Praise for
The pain

This is a superb book. It is what you would expect from three highly regarded and expert professionals who have a huge amount of experience in this field. It is not surprising that they have come up with a book of this calibre. Informative, practical and clear, it will have a transforming effect on those who live with chronic pain.

Professor Bruce Robinson, AM MD MSc FRACP
Dean of the Faculty of Medicine, University of Sydney

The Pain Book is an excellent guide to understanding the processes underlying the experience of pain and how it can be managed more effectively. Grounded in scientific research, it presents recent findings in a very accessible way. From conventional medical treatments to innovative psychological methods based on cognitive behaviour therapy and positive psychology, the strategies are explained in a very clear and practical way. I recommend this book to any person who is suffering from pain—you will never think about it in the same way again.

Dr Sarah Edelman, Clinical Psychologist and author, Change Your Thinking.

An outstanding book about living with the misery of chronic pain— written by three remarkable people who are specialists in this particular field. The Pain Book is informative, interesting and offers hope and relief to its readers.

Anne Deveson AO, Writer and Broadcaster

The Pain Book can be your lifeline to recovery. It is so simply and beautifully written that it was easy to become immersed and not be conscious you are grappling with the complexity of the mechanisms of pain. Take heart and have hope that pain can become like your shadow—there, but following, not leading your life. The Pain Book will help you find the courage, stamina and skills to retrain the nervous system and get your life back on track.

Elizabeth Carrigan, CEO, Australian Pain Management Association Inc. (APMA)

At last a book that embodies a new relationship between health service providers and people in pain. While many books purport to provide answers for people living with chronic pain, rarely do you find one that has true healing power. The Pain Book not only provides practical pathways for taking control of pain, but also bravely and respectfully speaks of the deeper and transformative journey that many people in pain travel.

Coralie Wales, PhD, Founder and President Chronic Pain Australia

the pain book

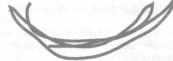

Finding hope when it hurts

HAMMOND
PRESS

PHILIP SIDDALL
REBECCA MCCABE
ROBIN MURRAY

Published by HammondPress
Sydney Australia
hammondpress@hammond.com.au
www.hammondcare.com.au

First published by HammondPress 2013.

10 9 8 7 6 5 4 3 2

Illustrations: Shalom Bourne. Cover and internal design: Melissa Summers.
Printed in Australia by SOS print+media.

ISBN: 978-0-9871892-7-1

National Library of Australia Cataloguing-in-Publications Data
Author: Siddall, Philip.
Title: The Pain Book: finding hope when it hurts/Philip Siddall, Rebecca McCabe,
Robin Murray; illustrations Shalom Bourne; design SD Creative; foreword Judith Lucy.
ISBN: 9780987189271 (paperback)
ISBN: 9780987582805 (ebook: epub); 9780987582812 (ebook: kindle)
Notes: Includes bibliographical references and index
Subjects: Chronic pain—Treatment. Chronic pain—Popular works.
Pain. Pain—Physiological aspects. Pain—Psychological aspects.
HammondCare. Greenwich Hospital.
Other Authors/Contributors: McCabe, Rebecca, author. Murray, Robin, author.
Bourne, Shalom, illustrator.
Dewy Number: 616.047

Dedication

Throughout this book, we hear from many people who tell their stories of pain. These are the voices of people we have seen in our own practice over many years.
Thank you for graciously telling your story.

We dedicate this book to you.

Contents

Foreword

I don't think you need to have pain of any kind to get something from this book.

The reality is, though, most of us are in pain. It may not be physical, or at least may not manifest that way. Whatever your experience, this book outlines ideas and strategies that are extremely useful when it comes to just living your life.

I should probably mention that I tend to be a little slow on the uptake when it comes to working stuff out. For a long time my way of dealing with pain or discomfort of any kind was to block it by annihilating myself. I was often filled with self-pity if not anger or hopelessness (no wonder I was single). It took me a long time to realise that life was about balance and it took decades before I worked out how important physical activity was to my wellbeing.

For me this activity happened to be yoga and this slowly led me to understand just how important is the connection between mind, body and spirit. Ultimately, that led me to making a series for the ABC called *Judith Lucy's Spiritual Journey* (where I was lucky enough to meet one of the authors of this book, Rebecca McCabe). As part of the show, I went on a 10-day silent meditation retreat and that's where I discovered how much my mind was like Mickey Rourke's face; a disturbing, inexplicable mess that I really needed to befriend.

The difficult part of the retreat, certainly for me, was not the silence or even the lack of shiraz, it was the pain I experienced from sitting in essentially the same position for more than 10 hours a day. After a few days, three hour-long sittings of 'strong determination'

> ' *This book offers a wonderful approach to pain management by suggesting we control what we can through knowledge and practical solutions.*'

were introduced during which we were very much encouraged not to move a muscle. My lower back was my issue and initially I focused so much on my discomfort that I honestly thought that I was going to have to approach one of the staff and request some sort of medical attention lest I wind up in a wheel chair. I am not exaggerating here. I really thought that I was doing irreparable damage to myself and of course the more I dwelt on it, the worse it became.

However, towards the end of the retreat, I was amazed at how quickly those hours flew by and by how little pain I now seemed to be experiencing. Nothing had changed apart from my approach. I no longer dwelt on the pain, I accepted it and not only that, during those days I had moments where I felt incredibly grateful, sometimes for nothing more than the sound of the rain, and this also led to a feeling of connection to something greater than myself.

This book offers a wonderful approach to pain management by suggesting we control what we can through knowledge and practical solutions. What I particularly love is the way it then encourages us to find hope and courage in our lives through the things we cannot control; by fostering gratitude, acceptance and by trying to find some sort of meaning—whatever that might be.

Good advice for dealing with pain and just a great way to live your life.

Judith Lucy

Introduction

Hope in the face of a hidden epidemic

Pain has been described as the hidden epidemic. One in five people suffer from chronic pain and so clearly it has a wide impact on our community. Behind the numbers is something that is often harder to see and that is the impact of pain on the individual. Chronic pain takes its toll on the body and it almost always affects the way a person thinks and feels. For many people, the impact of chronic pain is so deep and so strong that they lose hope that life will ever be the same again. For some, the effect is so overwhelming that they even question whether life is worth living.

In the face of such a problem, it is difficult to find hope. In the past few decades, some brilliant researchers have uncovered many of the mechanisms that underlie the experience of pain. As a result, new treatments are starting to flow through to the clinic and help many people with different types of pain. However, we still don't have the answer. For people with chronic pain, there is still no ready cure. What can we offer to the person who is living with chronic pain?

The answer lies in the pages of this book. The authors are all experts in the field. Philip Siddall is Professor in Pain Medicine at the University of Sydney with more than 30 years of clinical experience and international recognition for his research in this area. Rebecca McCabe is a physiotherapist with a special interest in chronic pain and many years experience in private practice and hospital pain management centres.

Robin Murray is a clinical psychologist who also has practised and taught in the field of pain management for many years in both hospitals and private practice. Together, they bring a breadth of knowledge and experience that is hard to equal.

This book provides an up to date overview of the latest understanding of how pain works as well as a summary of what is currently available for the treatment of pain. Above all, it provides a simple but effective step-by-step approach to treating pain using the most recent findings in the field of pain management.

This approach is based on the latest research. More than theory, the skills and techniques described in this book form the basis of a successful pain program run by the authors at Greenwich Hospital which is a teaching hospital of the University of Sydney managed by independent Christian charity, HammondCare. Careful evaluation of outcomes from this program tells us that people who put this approach into practice show significant improvements in how they think, how they feel and what they can do. In addition, their pain is reduced.

So, if you have pain, there is hope. There is hope that life can be better than it is right now. A life that contains less fear and more joy. A life that includes relationships and activities that bring satisfaction and pleasure. And a life that is free from the demands and control of pain. It is possible to face pain and to find hope when it hurts.

Part one
Facing pain

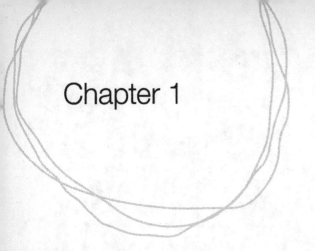

Chapter 1

Understanding pain

'The greater understanding we have of pain and how it works, the better equipped we are to manage it...'

Getting to know your pain

You may have heard it said that knowledge is power. In the case of dealing with pain, it is certainly true. The greater understanding we have of pain and how it works, the better equipped we are to manage it and the more sense of control we have over it. Time and time again, we see people who have had pain for many years but have little understanding of what it is or how it works. This adds to their sense of helplessness and frustration.

Everyone's pain is different. We will explore the various ways that pain can present and enable you to identify and understand your pain. We will delve into the latest information from scientific research that helps you understand what is happening in your body. And we will look at the impact of pain on the person as well as the treatments that are currently available.

Some of this may be familiar—much of it will almost certainly be new. It is based on the latest information we have available on understanding and treating pain. What is exciting is that recent research has uncovered important clues that hold wonderful promise for treating pain. These chapters are much more than information. They are the first steps in treating your pain.

Two main types of pain

Acute and chronic

Pain is usually divided into two main types according to how long it is present: acute and chronic. **Acute pain** is pain that lasts for a short time and is usually associated with damage or disease that can be treated. For example, pain from a fractured arm, burns, surgery, kidney stones or giving birth are all examples of acute pain. Once the fracture or wound is healed or the kidney stone is passed or the baby is born, the pain usually goes away.

Chronic (persistent) pain is pain that lasts for a long time. The definitions vary and the division can be a little artificial. However, in clinical practice, pain that lasts longer than three months is generally regarded as chronic. Chronic non-cancer pain can be due to many conditions, such as arthritis, migraine and tendonitis. It can also be due to nerve damage associated with conditions such as shingles, diabetes, trigeminal neuralgia and spinal cord injury.

Chronic pain may be ongoing but it is rarely felt at the same intensity all the time. For most people, the pain will vary according to what they do, how they feel and other factors such as the time of day or the weather. Most people also experience 'pain flares'. These are periods when the pain is more severe. Flare-ups can occur for a variety of reasons, such as changes in activity, travel, lack of sleep, stress or changes in hormones. Sometimes it won't be possible to identify anything particular that caused the increase in pain. Pain flare-ups can last from a few hours to a few weeks but do not necessarily signal a worsening problem. They can be a result of changes within the body, such as muscle spasm or inflammation, which increase pain temporarily but settle over time. But they can also be due to short term, reversible changes in the nervous system that temporarily amplify the messages coming from the area where you feel pain.

Chronic: the most challenging pain

Of the two types, chronic pain is usually more difficult to treat. Acute pain can be severe but it usually lessens as the tissue damage or injury heals. We also have fairly good ways of keeping it under control. On the other hand, it is often difficult to work out what is causing chronic pain, despite many investigations and visits to health professionals.

'Pain flare-ups can last from a few hours to a few weeks but do not necessarily signal a worsening problem.'

Even if a cause can be found, often there are no treatments that provide good relief. Treatments that do help may cause side effects that make life even more miserable. Therefore, chronic pain can prove the most challenging type to treat and people are often left frustrated, disappointed and hopeless.

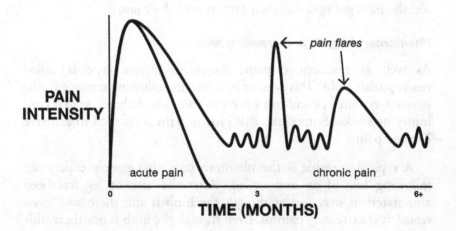

Cancer pain

Some people regard **cancer pain** as a specific type of pain but it can take many forms. Pain may occur from the spread of cancer into bones, pressure from a tumour on nerves or local pressure as a tumour expands. Although cancer pain is often feared, there are now many treatments that can keep it under reasonably good control.

The expert's perspective: Nociceptive and neuropathic pain

Health professionals also classify pain on the basis of where it is coming from and this generally falls into two major types. **Nociceptive pain** comes from two broad areas of the body. The first is **somatic pain** that comes from the skin, muscles, bones, joints and ligaments. Muscle, bone and joint pain is the most common type of chronic pain and referred to as **musculoskeletal pain**. It includes arthritis pain, most types of low back and neck pain and tendonitis. This type of pain can be dull and aching or localised and sharp. Musculoskeletal pain is usually made worse by movement and eased by rest. It often responds to treatments such as heat, anti-inflammatory medications, paracetamol and opioid medications such as morphine.

The second type of nociceptive pain is **visceral pain** which comes from the stomach and other organs in the abdomen. It includes pain such as appendicitis, kidney stones or a heart attack. It is usually dull and aching or cramping and difficult to localise. Visceral pain can also cause referred pain so that pain caused by a body organ is felt somewhere else. For example, people experiencing a heart attack may feel the pain going down their arm or into their jaw.

Phantoms, shingles and crawling ants

As well as nociceptive pain, the other major type is called **neuropathic pain**. This type of pain occurs following damage to the nervous system in conditions such as shingles, diabetes, spinal cord injury or stroke. Sometimes this type of pain is referred to as nerve damage pain.

A typical example is the phantom pain that people experience following loss of an arm or leg. After the arm or leg has been amputated, it may feel as though the limb is still there and, even worse, it is extremely painful. Even though the limb is not there, this pain is very real and is due to the damaged nerves sending signals back to the brain and causing the sensation of pain.

Another example is the pain that many people experience after an episode of shingles. Shingles is a condition that affects the nerves, where people get a rash, usually in a strip around the chest wall or another part of the body. Once the rash goes away, people can

'The skin can be extremely sensitive to touch so that even the wind or sheets touching the skin can cause severe pain.'

be left with numbness, tingling and terrible shooting and burning pain. Again, this is due to the damaged nerves sending messages that cause pain.

Neuropathic pain is often described as shooting, electric or burning and people often have abnormal sensation in the area surrounding their pain. The skin can be extremely sensitive to touch so that even the wind or sheets touching the skin can cause severe pain. Other people feel as though the skin has a numb feeling 'like cardboard' or they have a feeling of ants crawling under the skin. Neuropathic pain is not usually helped much by anti-inflammatory medications or even strong painkillers like morphine. However, it may be helped by more specialised treatments that we will discuss later (see page 43).

Some other pain conditions

Many chronic pain conditions cannot be neatly labelled as nociceptive or neuropathic. For example, many people with low back pain have a mixture of nociceptive pain caused by problems in the muscles and joints as well as neuropathic pain caused by a bulging disc irritating or pressing on nerves going down the leg (sciatica).

1 These and the following numbers throughout the book refer to articles that describe findings from research. If you are interested, these articles are listed at the back of the book.

There are also several other types of pain that are more difficult to group into these categories. These include conditions such as irritable bowel syndrome, fibromyalgia and complex regional pain syndrome. With irritable bowel syndrome, people get a mix of symptoms such as pain, diarrhoea, constipation and bloating but investigations usually find little if anything wrong with the stomach or bowel. With fibromyalgia, people report widespread muscle pain, tenderness and stiffness. Again there is little to find in the muscles that would seem to explain the severe pain.

Complex regional pain syndrome typically affects a whole arm or leg. It can occur after even the most minor trauma but people can have severe pain, weakness and the whole limb can change colour or temperature. Once again, although there is often a history of injury, the expected healing time is well past and there is little if any damage to find at the site of trauma.

If it's hurting, it's pain

Because it's difficult to find damage in these conditions, people are sometimes treated with scepticism and even labelled as neurotic. However, researchers have shown that the pain experienced may be due to an overactive or sensitised nervous system that amplifies messages coming from the site of pain.[1] Even though the messages coming from the bowel (in the case of irritable bowel syndrome) or the muscles (in the case of fibromyalgia) are not strong, the nervous system may be so sensitised that the messages are hugely amplified, resulting in ongoing pain. This means that the message is distorted or out of proportion to what is causing it, but is still very real.

Why the nervous system becomes so sensitised in some people is a matter that is being closely studied and we already have a few clues as to why this may be. What we have uncovered is that the way that we experience pain is due not only to what is happening in our bones, joints, muscles or organs but also the way that our nervous system registers and processes this information. This leads us into the next chapter where we will explore the fascinating insights that science has given us on how pain works and answer some of the questions about why we experience pain the way we do.

Fact File

- Everyone's pain is different.
- Chronic pain is very different from acute pain
- A sensitised nervous system may amplify pain.
- The more we know about pain, the better we can manage it.

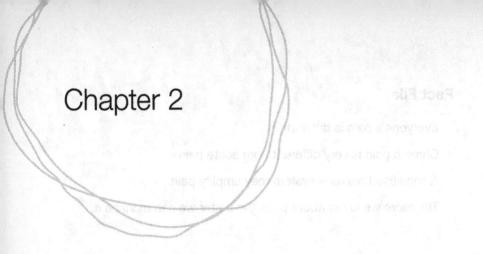

Chapter 2

How does pain work?

I was running late for my train and rushed down to the platform. Luckily it had just arrived and was coming into the station. But in my hurry to get onto the platform my foot caught on something just near the edge of the platform and I tripped. I fell toward the railway tracks. There was nothing I could do. As I looked up, I saw the train coming straight at me. It was all in slow motion. Then it hit me. The train went straight over one arm and nearly cut it off completely. But I didn't lose consciousness. I was awake the whole time. The weird thing was I knew everything that was happening to me. I could see my arm dangling but I didn't feel any pain the whole time.

Ben C, age 24, student

Unravelling the mystery of pain

As this story shows us, there are many things that we don't understand about pain. You may have heard of other similar stories. How is it that someone can go through an incident like this and not feel pain? Importantly, what can we learn from these sorts of experiences that might help us overcome pain?

Scientists have done a remarkable job in the past hundred years of helping us to unlock some of the secrets of pain. These findings have provided vital clues for treatment. In this chapter, we will look at what we know about how pain works: the way messages travel from the site of pain to the brain, the way that the brain controls the way we experience pain and the important link between pain and the mind.

Receiving the message: your receptors

The first step in our experience of pain is a stimulus, such as something hot or sharp, which stimulates **receptors** on our nerves.[1] These receptors are specially designed to react to a stimulus that may potentially harm us.

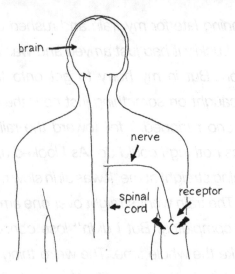

brain

nerve

spinal cord

receptor

For example, some of these receptors will only respond to temperatures above a certain limit (around 45OC) or only to certain chemicals such as acid.

Any time that receptors are stimulated by something that is potentially harmful, they very quickly start to send messages along the nerves toward the spinal cord, the main highway for information from the body to the brain. Nerves are found in nearly all parts of our body. They are found in the skin as well as many parts inside our body such as bones and joints and organs such as the heart and stomach.

The other process that occurs near the receptors that is extremely important in our experience of pain is **peripheral sensitisation**. Once a receptor on the skin surface or within the body is activated, it causes the release of chemicals that make the receptor even more sensitive. We can see this when joints get inflamed and go red or the skin goes red after a burn.

Peripheral sensitisation is important because it amplifies our experience of pain so that once something is inflamed, even the slightest movement or touch can result in pain. As we shall see later, anti-inflammatory drugs work by reducing inflammation and peripheral sensitisation and in this way reduce the pain.

Registering the message: your brain

Once a stimulus has activated the receptors, a message is sent along the nerve toward our spinal cord. In the spinal cord, these nerves enter and

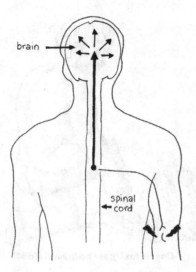

brain

spinal
cord

pass on the messages to the next relay, whose job it is to take information to the brain. The way that our brain processes these messages is a fascinating and complex process that has only recently begun to be understood.

People used to believe that there was a place in the brain that was specifically set apart for feeling pain, in the same way that there is a part of the brain for hearing and another one for seeing.

We now know the process is much more complicated and that pain messages go to many different parts of the brain. These different parts of the brain are involved in a whole range of processes. These include identifying where the message is coming from and what it is like, through to much more complex reactions such as fear, anger and the desire to escape.[2]

What is important for our experience of pain is that the brain does not just register that it is present. When the brain registers that a message is signalling pain, it responds. The brain sends messages back down the spinal cord that control blood pressure, heart rate, breathing and muscles. Most importantly, it sends messages that control the amount of information coming up the spinal cord, including pain information.

As we shall see, this connection between the brain and spinal cord that controls the amount of pain we experience is hugely important. It provides a way that we can tap into our nervous system to influence our own levels of pain. We will revisit this and see what it means for controlling our pain.

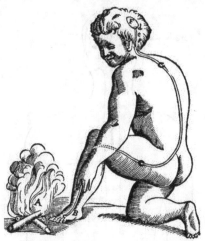

Descartes' 'pain pathway' (1664)

Do we all feel pain the same way?

For most of history, people have regarded pain as a message that simply warned us about damage. This means that we should all feel pain pretty much the same way. If there isn't much damage, the messages should be weak and we wouldn't expect to feel much pain. If there is a lot of damage, the messages should be strong and we could expect to have a lot of pain. So we should expect more pain from a broken leg than a sprained ankle, and two people with a broken leg should both experience the same amount of pain.

Actually, this is far from true. Pain is very different for everyone. It is true that what switches on the nerves is nearly the same for all of us. For example, nearly everyone has nerves that will switch on when they are heated to about 45°C and start sending messages toward the brain. Whether you are tall, short, Asian, Caucasian, African, male, female or even a chimpanzee, nerves respond in very similar ways.

However, when messages reach the spinal cord everything changes. By the time the brain gets hold of them, they will be even more different. Most of us have observed or even felt this fact ourselves. People playing sport can have severe injuries and not feel any pain. Even soldiers in battle can have terrible wounds and yet not feel much pain.[3] Pain is not that simple. As we heard in the story at the beginning of this chapter, a person can have a major injury but not experience much pain. On the other hand, some people have a minor injury and experience severe pain. The gate theory that was put forward in the 1960s helped us to understand why.

The gate theory: a breakthrough!

The gate theory was put forward by two leading researchers in 1965[4] and had a huge impact on the way that people saw pain. The gate theory proposed that pain messages coming into the spinal cord did not just go straight up to the brain.

Instead, it proposed (and there was evidence to support this) that there is a kind of gate in the spinal cord that controls the messages going up to the brain. This gate acts as a kind of volume control. It can be opened and the volume turned up so that we feel more pain. Or it can be closed and the volume turned down so that we feel less pain.

The gate or volume control in our spinal cord is an extremely important part of the pain experience because it means that the amount of pain we feel is not directly related to how much damage is present. If the gate is open and the volume turned up, the amount of damage may be small but the pain may be severe. On the other hand, if the gate is more closed, the pain may be minor even though the damage is major.

We also know that the brain helps to control the gate and the amount of information coming through. This is also important because it means through our brains we can control the amount of pain we experience.

What is the gate really like?

Even though we use the word 'gate', of course it is not a real gate in the spinal cord. In reality, there are very small nerve cells called inhibitory nerves whose job it is to block or filter information coming from different parts of our body. These cells are found in the spinal cord and the brain. In fact, we have many of these cells at every level of the spinal cord. They are also found in a part of the brain called the thalamus which is the main relay station that receives messages from the spinal cord and sends them on to different parts of the brain.

These inhibitory nerve cells in the spinal cord and brain help to regulate the amount of information that goes to the brain. You can imagine how many messages are coming from every part of our body at any one time. To name just a few, there is information about your last meal, your skin temperature, your breathing, the tightness of your clothes and the fullness of your bladder. If the brain had to process all of that information, it would go into overload! Unless they are particularly strong, most of the time we are only aware of many of these sensations when we consciously choose to focus on them.

This lack of awareness is because these inhibitory nerve cells constantly block or filter incoming information and allow the brain to focus on what it wants or needs to know about. It is these inhibitory neurons that create the gate. If they are switched on, they reduce the amount of information and 'close the gate'. If they are switched off, the gate is allowed to open.

So the 'gate' is a picture that we will use in this book to describe this inhibitory system in the spinal cord and brain. Even though it is a picture, it describes a real process that is going on in your nervous system all the time.

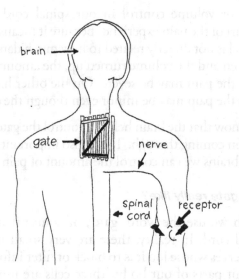

The gate and chronic pain

The state of the gate may help to explain why some people are more likely to experience certain chronic pain conditions. For example, we mentioned previously the condition called fibromyalgia, where people experience widespread pain in their muscles but there is little damage to find.

There is increasing evidence that people with this condition have a problem with their gate. It is not damaged but there is something happening in their brain that sends messages to open the gate and allow more messages to get through. This turns up the volume of the messages coming from the muscles so that pain is much stronger than would be expected.

The reason why some people have a gate that is abnormally open is not clear. It may be due to genetic factors that mean it is simply part of their makeup. Or it may be that previous experiences change the settings of the gate and leave it further open.

Whatever the reasons, it is now clear that the severity of pain is due not only to what is happening in the muscles but possibly even more so to what is happening in the spinal cord. That means that for many people with chronic pain, focusing on closing the gate is just as important, if not more important, than trying to fix something in the bones, joints, muscles or wherever the pain is coming from.

Opening the gate: increasing the volume

Knowing what opens and closes the gate (or turns up and down the volume—another useful word-picture) is extremely important in understanding the pain experience as well as in looking to what we can do to help reduce pain. Let's look at what opens the gate and first up, we know that our emotional state alters the gate. For example, it's more open when we are anxious or tense and we also know that lack of sleep can open the gate.

Unfortunately for people with chronic pain, pain itself opens the gate or turns up the volume. Incoming pain messages start a process that changes the volume control so that, as more pain messages come in, the volume is turned up and the pain is stronger.

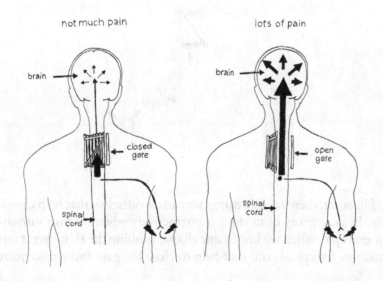

This is a process called **central sensitisation**.[5] If we have had pain for a while, our nervous system is sensitised. This means we are more sensitive to a stimulus coming from our body and feel more pain. The important thing to know is that for people with chronic pain, increased pain does not necessarily signal more damage. This sensitisation of the nervous system means that the pain can be strong even though the problem that caused your pain initially has settled or stabilised.

Closing the gate: turning down the volume

Although there are things that open the gate and increase our pain, there is a helpful side to the gate theory. A variety of things also close the gate or turn down the volume. If we can find out what helps close the gate, we can use this to reduce our pain. Many treatments work by closing the gate. For example, drugs such as morphine and antidepressants and stimulation techniques such as TENS, acupuncture and spinal stimulators help to close the gate and turn down the volume.

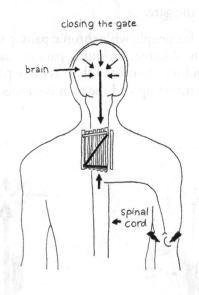

However, there are also things we can do ourselves that help close the gate. In fact, many of us do this instinctively when we hurt ourselves. For example, when we knock our elbow, rubbing the skin over it sends signals to the spinal cord that help to close the gate and reduce pain.

'Neuroplasticity simply refers to the fact that our nervous system is constantly changing.'

Our state of mind has a powerful influence on the gate and being relaxed or calm helps close it. Distraction can also have a strong effect on the gate and people who are absorbed in something can become almost oblivious to their pain.

The plastic nervous system

Our understanding of how the spinal cord and brain regulate pain and other messages by means of the gate, has revolutionised our view of pain and has huge implications for our ability to control it. However, there is another area of research that is not only fascinating but has had a major impact on how we understand pain - this is the field of neuroplasticity.

Neuroplasticity simply refers to the fact that our nervous system is constantly changing. It changes in response to injury, such as damage to nerves or the spinal cord, as the body tries to adapt and repair. Even if there is no injury, the brain will change if the messages coming from a particular part of the body increase or decrease. For example, most of us use an area of the brain called the sensory cortex when we touch an object and work out how sharp or cool or smooth it is. However, brain scanning has shown that when people who have lost their sight use their hands to assess an object, their visual cortex activates - the part of the brain normally reserved for making sense of what we see.

Another study looked at the brains of London taxi drivers who have to remember how to find their way through the vast numbers of roads and streets in London. Scientists found that for the taxi drivers, the part of the brain that helps to find places and remember where to go is much larger, compared with the rest of us. Again, it is a remarkable example of how the brain adapts or changes in response to what we do, what we think and the messages coming in from parts of our body.

Harnessing the power of neuroplasticity

We have looked at how neuroplasticity is a phenomenon that happens to our brains in response to something we do or something that happens to us. Although this is intriguing, so far it doesn't sound as though it is something that we have much control over.

The great news is that we can actually influence neuroplasticity ourselves and harness this phenomenon for our good. This is described beautifully in books such as *The Brain That Changes Itself* by Norman Doidge[6]. In this popular book, he tells the stories of people who have suffered from various conditions that have affected their nervous system. They then use findings from science to harness neuroplasticity, so regaining function and achieving amazing improvements in their quality of life.

One story is about a person who suffered a stroke resulting in extensive damage to the brain, with marked weakness on one side of the body and who is well past the point where further recovery would be expected. By continuing to work at specific exercises, they managed to improve and regain function in a way that was beyond expectations. Doidge attributes this to the amazing ability of the brain to adapt and compensate for damage by increasing the function of other parts of the brain. This shows there are things we can do that harness this ability of the nervous system to change and use neuroplasticity for our benefit.

Neuroplasticity and pain

Neuroplasticity is also extremely important in the experience of pain. Although it is still not clear whether pain is the result of neuroplasticity or the other way around, there is no doubt that neuroplasticity is present in people with pain.

If you have been in pain for any length of time, your nervous system, including your spinal cord and brain, has changed the way it functions. One of these changes we have already looked at in this chapter—central sensitisation. As we discussed, increased messages

'If you have been in pain for any length of time, your nervous system, including your spinal cord and brain, has changed the way it functions.'

coming from the area of pain makes the nerves in our spinal cord more sensitive and amplify our pain. This change in the way the nervous system functions is one type of neuroplasticity.

Pain is also linked to neuroplastic changes in the brain. Scientific studies have shown that pain is associated with a wide range of changes in the structure of the brain and the way that it works.

For example, the area of the brain that is mainly involved in sensation—the sensory cortex—is very neatly organised in a strip across the surface of the brain. This strip is like a map with each part of the sensory cortex representing different parts of the body. The area relating to the foot is near the middle of the brain and as you move along the brain surface you come to the legs, abdomen, chest, arms and head.

People with pain following an amputation (phantom limb pain) have a change in this map across the surface of the brain. The messages going to the part of the brain map that represent the hand and arm will obviously change following amputation. What's remarkable is that in people with pain, messages coming from the lip now also switch on the arm area of the brain map. Amazingly, this means that touching the lip in people who have phantom limb pain switches on the part of the brain normally reserved for registering messages from the missing arm.

So pain is linked to plastic changes in our brains and unfortunately these changes don't always seem to be helpful. Although neuroplasticity seems to be an adaptive response to help us recover from injury, in the case of pain it appears to be a maladaptive or unhelpful response.

Harnessing neuroplasticity to help pain

What we have described so far in terms of pain could sound quite negative. Although neuroplasticity is an amazing phenomenon, it doesn't sound very good for people with pain.

In fact, it is just the opposite. What we have learned about neuroplasticity offers tremendous hope for those with pain. Firstly, most of the evidence shows that these changes in the spinal cord and brain are reversible. For example, people with osteoarthritis pain have been shown to have shrinkage of some of the cells in one part of the brain. However, following a hip operation, these changes go away and the brain returns to normal. Similarly, central sensitisation in the spinal cord will settle once the pain is removed.

Secondly, even if we can't eradicate the pain, there are things that we can do that alter the way the brain and spinal cord function and so change the pain. Because the brain is plastic, our brains and our pain are not fixed. There are simple mental and physical techniques we can learn that harness the power of neuroplasticity to 'retrain the brain' and reset the nervous system, including the gate.

We are not saying that pain is all in your mind, nor that it is a question of 'mind over matter'. What we are saying is that your experience of pain is more than what is happening in your joint or your nerve or your disc or wherever your pain is coming from. We now know that it is also about what is happening in your spinal cord and brain. That means that if you have chronic pain, simply trying to fix the 'broken part' is unlikely to be the answer to curing your pain. On the other hand, no matter what is causing your pain, learning some simple skills that harness neuroplasticity can be powerful tools in helping to control your pain.

Can we control our pain with our minds?

I had to protect my inside self. Even though I suffered extreme pain my mind took over to protect me. I was tortured. I was stripped naked then placed on a metal bed. I was tied with wire to the bed and blindfolded.

'The view of pain as either real or psychological is simplistic and often unhelpful.'

> The wires were attached to different parts of my body and then they applied the current. The pain was indescribable, beyond my control. My mind protected me at the time from dying inside. I kept saying to myself it will end. I thought of how much I loved my wife and children. I tried not to think of the pain or the terrible people who were doing this to me.
>
> **MT, Afghani refugee, engineer, age 35**

Although the role of the brain or mind is clearly very significant, it can also be confusing.

In the past, many people thought of the role of the mind as being an all-or-nothing phenomenon. That meant that either the pain was all due to what was happening in the body or it was all due to what was happening in the mind. In other words, pain was real or it was psychological, and if it was psychological it was all in your head.

This view of pain is still around, and many people with pain may be dismissed by health professionals and others simply because the pain seems to be out of proportion to the damage. Although some people do have pain that is purely psychological, it is actually very rare.

In nearly all people who present with pain, there is something real that is giving rise to it. The view of pain as either real or psychological is simplistic and often unhelpful.

Good news: our brains make a difference!

Although pain is rarely just psychological, it is always influenced by how we think and feel because of the ability of the brain to close or open the gate. This is actually incredibly good news. It can be a force that we use to help ourselves. If we can change thoughts or feelings that are opening the gate or learn ways we can close the gate, we have something within our own grasp that will enable us to turn down the volume and control our pain.

Ben and MT's stories in this chapter illustrate the powerful ability of the mind to close the gate. They are remarkable examples of how the brain can block out pain. Even though it may seem dramatic, we too can tap in to some of these same mechanisms and learn skills that help our nervous system to close the gate and turn down the volume of our pain.

For example, something as simple as exercise can help to close the gate and reduce pain. Some people have learned mind skills that are so effective at blocking pain that they can have a needle stuck through their tongue and not feel pain. Amazingly, if you measure their brain activity and record what is happening while the needle is going through, there is nothing in their brain to indicate any pain.[7]

Not everyone can learn skills to this depth. However, it is abundantly clear that the brain not only registers pain but has a powerful influence on how much pain we experience.

This power of the brain to reduce pain can be switched on, not only by mind techniques, but also by simple things such as exercise and relaxation. This means that there is the potential for all of us to tap into this power to control pain and use the brain to our advantage.

As we shall see later, there are skills that anyone can learn that help close the gate and turn down the volume of pain. Learning these skills will not only help you feel better but will be a potent tool in reducing pain.

Fact File

- Scientists have unlocked some of the secrets of pain.

- Central sensitisation makes the nervous system more sensitive and amplifies pain.

- The amount of pain we feel may not be directly related to the amount of damage.

- Our brains don't just register pain, but also respond to it.

- Pain is rarely just psychological but it is always influenced by how we think and feel.

- We can retrain our brains to better control our pain.

Chapter 3

How does pain affect us?

Chronic pain is like throwing a stone into a lake of water. The stone is the pain and the ripples affect every part of your life.

Mary, age 55, solicitor

Pain: the gift that nobody wants

None of us like pain. It has been described as the gift that nobody wants. Acute pain is not pleasant but at least we can understand its purpose and usefulness and most of us are prepared to tolerate it from time to time.

It can be a very useful warning signal that alerts us to the fact that something is wrong. In fact, there are some people who have a very rare genetic condition that means they do not feel pain.[1][2] This may sound as though it would be very desirable. Sadly, however, these people suffer from major injuries that can even result in death. This is because their body has no way of communicating that there are problems that need to be taken care of.

Chronic pain is different. It seems to serve no useful purpose and continues despite the fact that we are well aware of the problem. Or it may even be present when there seems to be no problem at all. It is this ongoing pain and discomfort, which does not appear to be of any use and yet cannot be relieved, that makes living with chronic pain so hard.

The impact of pain

My response was to try and grin and bear it. Outwardly I was not saying much; inwardly I was screaming. Emotionally it never goes away. When you close your eyes it is there—when you open your eyes in the morning it is there. It is always there.

William, age 70, retired coal miner

Although it is helpful to understand how pain works, it is only half the issue.

It is not just pain itself but the impact of pain in our lives that is important. In fact, in some ways, the impact of pain can be worse than the pain itself. It is the effect of pain on our body, mind and spirit as well as on our activities and relationships that can wear us down, take away hope and remove pleasure from life.

The short-term impact of pain on our body

Pain is first and foremost a physical experience. Our body is highly programmed to react to pain in very defined ways. As the messages travel along nerves and reach the spinal cord, they first produce an automatic withdrawal response which is designed to remove the part of the body from whatever is causing pain. If our hand touches something that is sharp or hot, it will automatically withdraw even before we are conscious of the pain.

This response is so built in to our nervous system that we do not even need to be conscious to do it. People who are unconscious or even brain damaged will pull away if something or someone pinches their hand or foot. As the pain signals go higher up the spinal cord and reach the base of the brain, they trigger more complicated automatic reactions. Our blood pressure and heart rate go up and our rate of breathing increases. Then, as the signals go even higher, they trigger even more complicated emotions such as fear, escape and attack.

The long-term impact of pain on our body

Withdrawal from pain, tightening of muscles and other changes in heart rate and blood pressure occur within seconds of something causing us pain. So you can imagine the effect of constant pain on the body.

Even though our body adjusts, still it can result in long term changes. For example, as we have seen, the natural response to pain is to switch on muscles so that we withdraw and pull away. Even though we may not keep on withdrawing with chronic pain, pain can still send messages to the muscles so that they become tight and tense. This increased **muscle tension** can be the cause of more pain and make us even more uncomfortable.

Muscle tension can also add to our pain more indirectly by spreading to muscles in other areas and causing changes in posture which can further add to pain.

Over time, chronic pain can also lead to muscle weakening or de-conditioning. The natural inclination for anyone who is in severe pain is to avoid doing things such as bending, walking or lifting that seem to make the pain worse.

Our bodies are designed to move. When we decrease our activity levels, we lose muscle strength and become weaker and unfit. Over time this loss of strength affects our independence and even simple activities of daily living such as getting out of a chair and walking can become increasingly difficult.

This **physical deconditioning** can cause more problems. It can indirectly add to the pain by contributing to postural problems and producing more pain messages. Unfortunately, when we are not moving or exercising, we don't produce the naturally occurring chemicals in our bodies called endorphins that close the gate and turn down the volume of pain.

Trevor's story

As well as affecting the body, pain has a huge impact on how we feel. Trevor's story is similar to those of many others who have chronic pain and illustrates the impact of pain on the mind as well as the body.

Trevor presented to the Pain Management Centre with pain in the neck, arms, chest and hips after something fell on his head and partially damaged his spinal cord. Fortunately, the damage to the spinal cord was not severe and Trevor could still walk and continue his job managing a successful business.

However, although he recovered well in terms of function, he was left with severe neuropathic pain that was related to the damage to his spinal cord and nerves.

We tried the usual treatments for neuropathic pain, including antiepileptic drugs and antidepressants, and they helped, but only a little. He had constant stinging and burning pain that made it difficult to work and difficult to sleep. He was tired, irritable and depressed and all of this was interfering with his relationships with his wife and children.

Some time after starting treatment, Trevor sent the following note to describe how he felt. He titled it *Life*.

Life

It's Sunday and I'm at work feeling sorry for myself.

The pain levels have been very high for such a long time now that I feel totally worn out and don't know how to escape the problem pain I'm in, not that I ever have.

It is a real bitch.

I feel like I'm drugged and life is like a dream.

How does one get out of this?

I'm in agony and no one can tell.

It just tells me I do a good job of getting through the days.

But what am I to do, my arms are stinging off the wall, I feel like I have broken ribs and my hips have now been killing me for months and sleep is a real s***.

I keep my mouth shut but only feel like screaming my lungs out that the pain is overwhelming me.

The years have passed and I didn't think I would last the first year, yet I fear, will this be the year I give up.

One gets so tired of the fight that you can't help but think of giving up.

I often think of taking a long rest with no more pain and the thoughts feel good to dream of it ending.

Some days are just a complete bitch where you try to distract yourself but can't.

How much can one person take?

It is a very interesting question because I'm still here, waiting for the fateful day my armour cracks.

Trevor

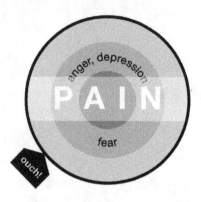

The impact of pain on our mind

Unfortunately Trevor's story and the feelings he describes are not unusual. Many people with pain share these feelings of tiredness, frustration, hopelessness and being overwhelmed and yet also show similar courage and determination.

As well as these feelings, people also struggle with other emotions such as **anxiety** and **fear**. People in pain soon learn that some things they do bring on pain and so they avoid these situations for fear of causing pain or making their pain worse. They can be fearful not only about experiencing the pain, but also about what the pain means, whether something has been missed, and what the pain means for their future and their relationships.

Pain also causes **depression**. Depression comes from living constantly in pain and discomfort and the way that this takes away pleasure from life. It is made worse by loss of other things such as work, activities and relationships that used to bring satisfaction and enjoyment. These losses can result in grief and sadness.

I found that chronic pain and occasional flare-ups to what was an unbearable level of pain could play on my mind so much that the fear and anxiety this produced made it difficult to relax or enjoy life.

Pain can also result in **anger** at others or even ourselves for getting us into this situation or not being able to get out of it. This anger can bubble out of control and be expressed at employers and doctors and even those who are close to us such as family members and friends. This can happen even though we can sometimes see that it is unreasonable or undeserved.

Of course, the mind and body are closely related and the effects on one spill over to the other. Physical inactivity and deconditioning can add to depression. Anger can lead to further increases in muscle tension. Withdrawal and avoidance lead to further lack of activity and deconditioning. These effects on mind and body combine and interact to make the pain experience worse.

The impact of the mind on our pain

I developed lower back pain after my second child. I went to the GP, he did some investigations and told me I had a slipped disc. I was 29-years-old. I immediately stopped my aerobic classes because that made my pain worse. I thought if I keep going the disc that had slipped could slip right out! I was terrified to think of what could happen to me in the future. I thought if I am like this at 29 what am I going to be like at 69! I became depressed and angry. My weight ballooned to 80kg. After about eight months I went back to my GP. She sent me for an X-ray and reassured me that my disc hadn't deteriorated. She also said that increases in my pain didn't mean more damage to my disc in my back. The pain from my back in fact was not telling me any more information than I already knew. I can't tell you what a difference that advice made to my life. My mind stopped racing to the worst possible scenarios. I am back doing aerobics, back at work and have three children.

Robin, age 48, accountant

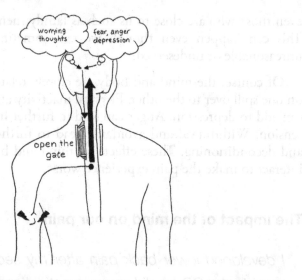

Pain not only affects our mind, but the state of our mind can greatly affect our pain. In the last chapter, we saw the close link between the mind and its ability to influence the gate and turn up our pain. We now know that negative thoughts and emotions can feed back and add further to the volume of the pain.

Depression can add to a process called **catastrophising**. Like Robin, whose story we have just heard, people can tend to think the worst is going to happen. For example, if they have back pain and they know they have a disc problem, they may think that they are in real danger of becoming paralysed and ending up in a wheelchair, even though they have been told that everything is stable. Catastrophising is not just unpleasant, it directly makes our experience of pain stronger.

Another process linked to catastrophising is **hypervigilance**. Hypervigilance is a situation where our bodies and minds become finely attuned to what is happening around them – inside the body as well as out. All of us have a sort of internal radar that is constantly spinning and picking up information from inside our body and the world around us. When we are anxious or fearful, the radar starts spinning more vigorously so that we become much more aware of what is happening and much more sensitive to any sort of stimulus.

Hypervigilance and catastrophising are mental processes but they make the pain worse by switching on pathways that open the gate in the spinal cord, turning up the volume. These powerful processes link our mind to our body and add to pain.

The wider impact of pain

I just couldn't get away from my pain. It was like a demanding child wanting attention continuously. I was sensitive to all different pains in my body but I also became very sensitive to noise, light and heat. I used to enjoy going up to the local shopping centre for a coffee with friends but I found the noise, light, and crowded places made my pain worse. I was exhausted most of the time. I became my pain and I lost everything—my husband, my children, my work, myself.

Julie, age 36, hairdresser

Julie's story shows us that pain can have an overwhelming impact on our mind and deeply affect our thoughts and emotions. However, it is not just the pain but the other circumstances that surround chronic pain that can also contribute to how we feel.

The ongoing desperate search for something to make the pain better can actually cause more problems. Even in the best hands, many treatments such as medications or surgery can cause side effects and even make the pain worse. Many people with chronic pain suffer other losses. They may lose their jobs and as a result, lose contact with colleagues and workmates. It also means loss of income and sometimes becoming involved in disputes involving insurance companies, employers and lawyers. Pain also means loss of hobbies and sports that used to be fun and a way of keeping fit and active. Pain may also stop us spending time and enjoying activities with friends and family.

All of these things and more happen to people with chronic pain. And all of them have an impact. They can contribute further to negative feelings and thoughts and add to the cycle of pain.

The deeper impact of pain

These feelings and thoughts may go deeper. Fear of causing further pain can become a dominant factor in our lives, leading us to gradually withdraw from our usual way of life.

Anger may grow so that it starts to affect nearly everything we do. It not only deepens inside us but bubbles over and damages our relationships with people around us. We lose access to activities and relationships that we enjoy, and then face the further loss of pleasure or caring for anything. This may result in a deep bitterness and a hardening of spirit.

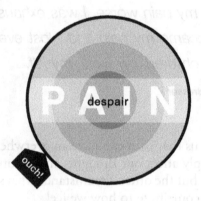

Depression may develop so severely that we become withdrawn, our world shrinks around us and it becomes even more centred on us and our pain. Pain dominates our present and our future and we become convinced that there is little to look forward to in life. Finally, we may lose any sense of hope and purpose and reach a point of **despair**.

The end result is that these feelings of despair may reach to the core of who we are. We feel as though we are no longer the person we used to be. Our spirit can be diminished or even crushed. Whereas once we had things in our lives that gave us meaning, purpose and enjoyment, we now feel worn out, hopeless and with little energy. We may even lose the will to live.

Pain has an impact that can affect the core of who we are – our spirit. We know from experience that people with persistent physical pain often face issues of grief and loss of meaning in life similar to those facing the end of life.

'Pain has an impact that can affect the core of who we are – our spirit.'

Research now being carried out in this area uses several tools to measure what is referred to as 'spiritual wellbeing' or its opposite, 'spiritual distress'. These tools evaluate aspects of a person's life such as their sense of hope, meaning and purpose. Many—but not all—people with terminal conditions such as cancer or HIV/AIDS show increased levels of spiritual distress. What is possibly surprising to some is that people with chronic pain have levels of spiritual distress that on average are even higher than people with cancer and HIV/AIDS.

Chronic pain: a source of grief, bitterness and despair

We have considered how pain works, how it affects us and learned that there are some positive and negative dimensions.

On the positive side, acute pain is an important and helpful warning sign that lets us know if some part of our body is damaged or in danger of being damaged.

On the negative side, chronic pain no longer functions as a good warning sign and hurts in many ways and at many levels. It results in physical effects such as muscle tension and deconditioning, which can feed back and add to our pain.

Pain also has emotional effects and leads to fear, anger and depression. Again, these effects can feed back and worsen pain by opening the gate and turning up the volume. Pain can affect us so deeply that we experience bitterness and despair.

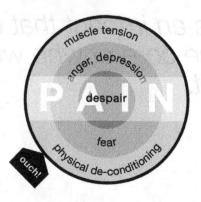

Living with pain in a way that makes life enjoyable again means addressing all of these secondary effects of having persistent pain. It means tackling the pain and reducing it as much as possible.

But it also means dealing with muscle tension, deconditioning, anger and depression. It means finding ways to deal with despair. If these things are addressed well, they will not only help us feel better but will also break the vicious cycle that is worsening the pain.

There is good news

The good news is that we do have ways of doing this.

As we have seen, the body has a powerful system in our brain and spinal cord to block out and control pain and this system is influenced by what we do, think and feel. This means if we can learn to modify our actions, thoughts and feelings, we can not only feel better and do more but we can actually reduce our pain.

This is what you will find in the next section of this book. We will give you skills that will help you become more active and relaxed, less fearful, angry and depressed and make life more hopeful and enjoyable. In the process, these skills will also help reduce your pain.

Before we do that though, it is good to make sure that you know what treatment is available and have considered all the options that may help.

Fact File

- Pain may impact our minds bringing anxiety, fear, anger and even depression

- Certain feelings such as anxiety may increase pain

- Certain ways of thinking such as catastrophising and hypervigilance may increase our pain

- Learning to change the way we think and feel may reduce our pain

- Taking control over our pain will make life more enjoyable.

Chapter 4

Good news: we can treat pain

It's time for some good news. If you have chronic pain, there is a reasonable chance that, although it may not be possible to get rid of the pain, it may be possible to provide a certain amount of relief. And if it is not possible to relieve it entirely, it is certainly possible to deal with its effects.

The job of any health professional you see about your pain, after they have figured out what they think is causing it, is to work out what be done to relieve it. As we shall see in this chapter, there is a whole range of approaches that can be used to relieve pain.

The skill of the health practitioner lies in accurate diagnosis so that the right treatment can be used. It is important to find someone whom you respect and trust to deal with your pain expertly and sympathetically so that they can apply the right treatment.

Who can help you?

Doctors

Of course, every doctor deals with people in pain. General practitioners (GPs) are usually the first port of call and if it is the first time that you present with this pain, the general practitioner will ask questions, perform an examination and perhaps order tests to try and work out what is causing it.

If the GP wants a further opinion or feels that specialised treatment is needed, you may be referred to a medical specialist. The type of specialist will depend on the problem you have. For example, if you have a persistent headache, they may send you to a neurologist or if you have knee pain they may send you to a rheumatologist or an orthopaedic surgeon.

Other health practitioners

In addition to doctors, there are a large number of other health professionals such as physiotherapists, chiropractors, osteopaths and others for whom much of their practice is focused on treating people with pain. These people often have a specialist interest, skills and qualifications and can be helpful in addressing certain problems and types of pain.

Pain clinics

Fortunately, most pain conditions resolve themselves or respond well to treatment. However, we know that one in five people have pain that continues despite treatment and the pain is then labelled as chronic.

In this case, general practitioners or other specialists may seek the advice of a Pain Clinic or Pain Management Centre. This is not always necessary but may be helpful if the local doctor or specialist would like further advice or specialised treatment.

Pain clinics have a team of professionals including doctors, physiotherapists, nurses, clinical psychologists and other health professionals who work together to treat people with chronic pain. These pain clinics are also staffed by pain medicine specialists who are specifically trained to deal with the issues involved.

How do health professionals help?

Drug treatment

All these people use a range of options for dealing with pain. Drugs are probably the most common way that people manage it. There are a number of pain-treating drugs available over the counter or on prescription. These drugs include analgesics such as paracetamol (Panadol or Dymadon among others), anti-inflammatory medications such as ibuprofen (Brufen, Advil, Nurofen) or naproxen (Naprosyn, Naprogesic, Aleve) and strong painkillers or opioids such as codeine, morphine and oxycodone.

As mentioned before, there are two main types of pain: nociceptive pain (which includes musculoskeletal and visceral) and neuropathic pain. These different types of pain respond differently to medications. Musculoskeletal pain such as arthritis or muscle pain and visceral pain such as period pain respond fairly well to **analgesics** and **non-steroidal anti-inflammatory drugs**. These drugs reduce the inflammation and peripheral sensitisation that we looked at earlier.

If the pain is acute and severe, such as with kidney stones or a fractured limb, strong painkillers such as morphine may be required. However, even in these cases, it is usually possible to make a person reasonably comfortable.

Sometimes, if you have severe chronic pain from muscles or joints, your doctor may feel that it is best to use a strong painkiller such as morphine or oxycodone. If this is the case, it is preferable to use preparations that are long acting, such as specially formulated tablets or patches. These preparations are more convenient and give a more stable level of pain relief throughout the day.

Neuropathic pain drugs

On the other hand, **neuropathic pain** is quite different from musculoskeletal pain and responds poorly even to high doses of strong painkillers such as morphine. This is because many of the mechanisms causing the pain are different. Musculoskeletal pain is largely due to messages being sent from a site of damage or disease. For example, if you have an arthritic hip, the joint can become inflamed and messages are sent to the brain so that pain is registered. Neuropathic pain is due to abnormal messages coming from the actual wiring, that is, from the nerves or spinal cord. This means that different drugs are used to target nerve and spinal cord changes.

Several types of different drugs targeting the nervous system are used. These include **antiepileptic drugs** such as gabapentin, pregabalin, carbamazepine (Tegretol, Teril) and valproate (Epilim, Valpro, Valprease). Although mainly designed for the treatment of epilepsy, these drugs work in neuropathic pain by dampening down the activity of nerves that send off messages when they are damaged.

The other group of drugs that are commonly used for treating neuropathic pain are the **antidepressants**. These are given not because your doctor may feel you are depressed but because they work by boosting chemicals in the nervous system that close the gate and block out pain. They are, therefore, working directly to reduce pain. If antiepileptics and antidepressants do not work, sometimes your doctor may add a strong painkiller. However, it typically only takes the edge off the pain and the body quickly becomes used to it so you need higher and higher doses to get the same effect.

Medications: the upside and the downside

Using medications is such a large part of pain management that it will be helpful to spend a little time here talking more about their use. Medications certainly have benefits. Particularly with acute pain, they can be very effective in relieving pain. Some specialised medicines for conditions such as neuropathic pain can also be very effective for some people—they have an important place in dealing with pain.

Medications can also have a downside. For many people with chronic pain, most medications provide only partial relief. Even this relief can lessen over time, particularly with medications such as opioid drugs like morphine or oxycodone. In addition, many medications have side effects. Although most side effects may not be serious, they can add problems like drowsiness, clouded thinking, constipation and stomach upset. This can make life more difficult and interfere with activities like work or driving.

The list of side effects is not meant to scare you. However, it is important to be aware that pain relief often comes at a price. That price should always be considered in trying to optimise the amount of pain you are prepared to accept and balance this against the negative effects of trying to reduce it. Ask your doctor or your pharmacist about what sort of side effects—both short and long term—you may experience. Also take the medication in the way it has been prescribed by your doctor. Don't be tempted to take more when you feel bad. Overusing medications can have serious side effects.

I was diagnosed with peripheral neuropathy in both legs four years ago. The damage to my nerves causes various painful sensations—burning in the soles of my feet, electric-like sharp jabs into my toes and extreme sensitivity to touch from my knees down. Over the last years I have tried many different pain medications and seen many doctors. I could write a book about the side effects of most pain medications! In my frantic search to stop the pain I hoped that someone would prescribe me a 'pill' that would stop my nerves firing and take the pain away. At one stage I was on five different medications for pain and depression. My wife asked me if they were working and my response was—I don't know—I still

'Pain relief often comes at a price. That price should always be considered in trying to optimise the amount of pain you are prepared to accept and balance this against the negative effects of trying to reduce it.'

have pain. I think I have the right mix now. I take two medications for my neuropathy which take the edge off my pain but don't 'bomb me out'! Medications help but are not a panacea. I have to do my bit as well—keep active, watch my diet and pace my activities.

John, age 72, retired policeman, father and grandfather

In summary, medications can be a useful part of helping to manage your pain. However, be wary of relying on them alone. If you do take medications, you will get the most benefit and keep the side effects to a minimum if you use them as part of a plan that includes other approaches.

Physical treatments

As well as medications, many people use physical treatments to manage their pain. Physical treatments may be particularly helpful for musculoskeletal pain and are done by people such as physiotherapists, occupational therapists, osteopaths and chiropractors.

Treatments include passive techniques such as **massage, interferential** and **transcutaneous electrical nerve stimulation (TENS)** and more active treatments such as **exercise programs** and

> *'The state of our mind has a huge influence on our experience of pain.'*

exercise techniques. However, the effect in chronic pain conditions, particularly for passive treatments may be fairly short term.

Active exercise that you can do and build into your lifestyle may be beneficial in correcting postural problems from disuse, reversing the deconditioning that can occur with chronic pain and rebuilding physical strength, which has a protective effect against worsening pain.

Psychological treatments

As mentioned previously, the state of our mind has a huge influence on our experience of pain, and pain itself has a large impact on our thinking and the way we feel. Therefore, particularly in those who have chronic pain, input from a clinical psychologist or psychiatrist may be very helpful in dealing with both the pain and its impact.

Some people are concerned that psychologists and psychiatrists just tell people that pain is all in their heads. However, their role is not to work out whether your pain is 'psychological' but to assess how pain is affecting your mood and to see how you deal with the pain. They can identify whether there are other issues such as major depression that may need treatment with psychological approaches or sometimes with medication. They can also examine the ways that you think about pain and structure your activities and suggest changes that help to reduce the pain and its impact on your life.

One of the approaches that clinical psychologists use is called **cognitive behavioural therapy (CBT)**. This is often done in groups

'Psychological treatment also focuses on how pain impacts on your relationships with others...'

and many pain clinics will run these programs either intensively over several weeks or in shorter sessions extended over a longer period.

The content of these programs vary. However, the aim is to reduce the impact that pain is having in your life and to help change your lifestyle so that you can return to activities that you enjoy. This can be done through physical exercise instruction, helping you to change the way you think about pain and guidance on how you structure your activities. Psychological treatment also focuses on how pain impacts on your relationships with others and addresses a host of other factors that can be helpful in returning to a more normal lifestyle.

Surgical treatments

Surgical approaches to pain have been used for many years. They can be very useful in situations such as osteoarthritis of the knee or hip. For example, **joint replacement** can result in a tremendous improvement in mobility as well as reduction in pain.

However, the outcomes in more complex conditions such as low back pain may be less successful. There is also evidence that the outcome of **back surgery** worsens with repeated procedures. If you have had back pain and previous surgery, the likelihood of improvement decreases with each operation. Although clearly indicated in some conditions where there is back pain, pain itself is not generally a good reason for surgery and back surgery should only be considered with a great degree of caution and following sound advice.

Beware of hunting for a surgeon who is prepared to operate on your back, because you may eventually find one!

Although the outcomes for joint replacement can be good and the results for back surgery variable, the outcomes for surgical treatment of neuropathic pain are almost always disappointing. If you have pain due to nerve damage, **cutting the nerve** or even the spinal cord is not the answer. For example, some people with neuropathic pain are so desperate to get relief that they consider amputation to get rid of the pain. Unfortunately, there are people who have done this and the pain almost always returns. Sadly, in some cases, the new pain is worse than the old pain.

Similarly, some people have all their teeth removed to try and remove pain in the jaw. Unfortunately again, they end up with no teeth but still the same pain.

Stimulation treatments

Another approach to treating pain is the use of stimulation techniques. These include techniques such as **transcutaneous electrical nerve stimulation (TENS), acupuncture, spinal cord stimulators, motor cortex stimulation** and even **deep brain stimulation**, which involves implanting electrodes deep into the brain. All of the stimulation techniques work by stimulating nerves and sending electrical impulses toward the spinal cord and brain. Many of these techniques act by releasing chemicals and closing the gate in either the spinal cord or the brain.

The evidence for stimulation techniques is not as strong as some other methods of relieving pain but some people find them effective for some conditions. Some stimulation techniques such as **TENS** have the advantage of being non-invasive and having minimal side effects. It is usually possible to organise a trial of these machines before purchasing, to see how much benefit they provide.

Acupuncture, of course, has been used for thousands of years and is now regarded in many quarters as mainstream medicine. There is good evidence from scientific studies that it has an analgesic effect by releasing pain chemicals and blocking pain. There is also evidence from a number of clinical studies that it may be helpful in some conditions such as osteoarthritis, headaches and fibromyalgia. It may also be helpful for problems such as neck pain and low back pain although the effect may be fairly short term.

'Beware of hunting for a surgeon who is prepared to operate on your back, because you may eventually find one!'

Implantable **spinal cord stimulators** may be useful, particularly for some types of neuropathic pain in the legs and complex regional pain syndromes. However, they are invasive and should only be considered after careful assessment in a Pain Management Centre where doctors can consider your pain condition and whether you are likely to receive benefit. **Deep brain stimulation** is very invasive and only done in a small number of centres. It can have serious side effects and there is limited evidence of its effectiveness.

Anaesthetic procedures

Anaesthetic procedures include techniques such as injections of local anaesthetics and steroids. These can be done into joints or nerves or around the spinal cord to block out pain. **Local anaesthetics** can be given this way and often provide very good relief of pain. However, the effect is temporary and so the usefulness for the treatment of chronic pain is more limited. Sometimes **steroids** can be injected around joints, nerves and the spinal cord and this can relieve pain by reducing inflammation. Again, however, the effect is fairly short term and repeated injections of steroids can have other effects that are best avoided.

A more long-lasting procedure that can be done is **radiofrequency lesioning**. This applies an electrical current through the end of a needle to lesion a small nerve that, for example, goes to a small joint in the spine. This can be very effective at relieving some types of back pain by removing the nerve supply and relieving the pain coming from that joint. Although it does disrupt the nerve, the effect appears to be limited to removing the pain with no other side effects. The nerve also appears to heal so that it is not a permanent lesion. This does mean though that the pain usually returns some months later. However, the procedure can be repeated.

Complementary and alternative approaches

A large number of people now use complementary and alternative therapies as part of managing their pain. Although there is some disagreement about what is regarded as conventional and what is regarded as alternative, they include treatments such as herbs, homeopathic remedies, naturopathy, aromatherapy, yoga, meditation techniques and acupuncture.

Many of these practices have their origins in religious traditions and philosophies and often the principles behind them and the way they are used are based on these traditions. They often have spiritual connections and people find they provide an added dimension that goes beyond the physical and emotional. They experience a connection to something deeper or bigger than themselves that provides a transcendent or even sacred aspect to the treatment.

It is not possible to give the evidence for all of these techniques and if you are interested in any particular treatment you may be able to find out specific information about it through a health professional or on good quality websites. However, a growing number of these practices have been subjected to scientific studies and show benefits for helping pain, as well as helping other aspects of our physical and emotional wellbeing. This means that they do have a place.

Having said that, the evidence for the effectiveness of some of these treatments is not strong. Some people find them helpful in that they provide a dimension that other conventional treatments don't provide. We would recommend discussing a treatment that you are considering with a health professional who is knowledgeable in that area. Try to get a realistic picture of the likely benefit and, as with any treatment, weigh this up against the cost and potential side effects.

We would recommend a balanced approach to the use of complementary and alternative approaches to pain. They are rarely the answer. However, as we shall explore later in this book, various alternative approaches can be useful in helping the body and mind and improving the pain. As long as we understand the limitations of these techniques as well as the benefits, they may be helpful tools.

'For most people with chronic pain, the main aim of treatment shifts from fixing the pain to managing the pain.'

What are these treatments trying to achieve?

Fixing the pain

Having described many of the treatments that are available for treating chronic pain, it is useful to ask the question: What are they trying to achieve? The answer to this question may sound obvious. However, there may be a big difference between what they are capable of doing and what the person receiving them thinks they are doing.

The first aim in treating pain is to identify the cause of the pain in the hope that the cause can be treated and that the pain goes away. For acute pain, this is generally possible. For example, we can see a kidney stone on an X-ray and removing it will result in relieving the pain. Or we can see a bone fracture on X-ray and putting on a cast or splint will help the bone to heal and the pain to go away.

With chronic pain, however, this may not be so easy. In many cases, such as nerve damage, we may be able to find out exactly what is causing the pain but have little ability to fix it. In other cases, we may simply be unable to say with any certainty what is causing the pain. For example, in many people with chronic back pain, it is impossible to determine exactly what structure is causing the pain. The chances of finding a cure then, are unlikely. In these situations, the person who continues to search for an answer to what is causing the pain in hope of a cure is on a frustrating and often expensive mission.

It is important to try and find out what is causing the pain. But if someone has been thoroughly investigated by those they trust and who know what the problem is but can't fix it, then it is important to move on from seeking a cure.

Managing the pain

For most people with chronic pain, the main aim of treatment shifts from fixing the pain to managing the pain. Managing can include relieving pain through to learning how to cope with pain. The emphasis on relief tends to vary in different situations. For example, for people with cancer pain, health practitioners may be much more willing to consider options such as large doses of strong painkillers like morphine or invasive treatments. This is because the benefit may outweigh the side effects as the person may not be expected to live very long.

However, in people who are expected to live a long time, health practitioners may be much more wary about certain options such as strong pain killers or surgical procedures. This is due to the possible further damage caused by surgery or the fear of addiction or tolerance with opioids. Tolerance occurs when the body becomes used to the medication and a person then requires higher and higher doses to sustain the same effect.

The other problem facing the search for pain relief is that it is often very difficult to get complete or even very good relief. This can mean that some people seek out more and more treatments in the hope that they will find one that will take away most, if not all, of their pain. Apart from being time-consuming and costly, these treatments often bring their own problems. For example, many people have major surgery and are extremely disappointed when their pain is not only still present but even worse following the operation.

A skiing accident in 2009 left me with a badly fractured right ankle. I had surgery to put my broken bones back together, was put in plaster for six weeks and then referred to a physiotherapist for four weeks rehabilitation. I was told the operation was successful and that I would be back to normal activities by three months. I did all my exercises diligently and did not miss an appointment. At three months I was still in considerable pain and on pain killers. I had MRI's, bone scans, blood tests, nerve conduction studies which did not show that much. I went on a search for a cure—conventional and alternative. I was 21 and in my third year of mechanical engineering. I tried everything from magnets to medications and spent money that I didn't have. I was desperate and therefore vulnerable to anyone that offered me a cure or a fix. I am now sure that this desperate search to stop the pain actually made the pain worse. I became angry, frustrated and depressed. I felt helpless and lost hope. Fortunately my local GP told me it was time to change tack. He encouraged me to step off the medical and alternate therapy merry-go-round. He took the time to explain why I still had pain even though the bones in my ankle had healed. He talked about the pain gate in my spinal cord. I found a physiotherapist who understood these mechanisms and helped me in stages to walk normally again. Through hard work, perseverance and a good dose of acceptance, my pain is reduced, I finished my studies and I am saving money!

Susan, age 28, engineer

Other people take steadily increasing doses of drugs in the hope that they will reach a point where they feel comfortable but are disappointed that the drugs merely take the edge off their pain.

A difficult message

When everything has been tried or at least considered, managing the pain is the line that many pain clinics are left to sell. It is a hard message to give someone. Understandably, people in pain want to hear that something can be done to take away their pain. Health practitioners treating pain understandably want to make people better.

However, if getting rid of the pain becomes the priority whatever the cost, the cost can become high. People can end up on an endless journey trying to find something or someone who will take away their pain. Health practitioners can feel forced into offering treatments that are expensive and have significant side effects, even though there is little evidence to support their use.

In these situations, coming to a point where a person recognises the need to manage the pain rather than try to fix it can be extremely important. Of course, it is vital that appropriate investigations are done to find the cause of the pain and that appropriate treatments are trialled. However, if this has been done and it appears that nothing is likely to take away the pain, then it may be time to move on.

It must be remembered that moving to management does not mean giving up on relief or even finding a cure. As we shall see, there are ways of managing your pain that do not just mean coping with what you have but actually reducing it. And it never rules out the possibility that a cure is somewhere down the line. The difference is in a shift of focus from fixing the pain to managing the pain.

The difficult question for many people is when to come to this point of shifting their focus. A suggestion would be that if your local doctor is satisfied that nothing further can be done, then it is time to shift. If for some reason you are not entirely happy with this decision, then a visit to a specialist or a pain clinic may be a useful further opinion. However, if they agree with your local doctor that nothing further can be done, then it is definitely time to change tack.

Is there an alternative approach to pain?

The approaches we've described so far are those currently suggested for the management of pain. The question is: How well do these approaches work?

There is no doubt that, as Ambroise Paré suggested all those years ago, cure and relief are our two top priorities in treating pain. Whatever else follows in the rest of this book, it needs to be quite clear that the first priority for any person with pain is to work out as far as is possible what is causing the pain. There may come a point where further attempts to define the source of the pain are unlikely to be helpful. However, it cannot be stressed enough that treating someone or telling someone to manage their pain without a reasonable idea of the cause or a good attempt to find it is poor medicine.

The relief of pain is also a high priority although, as we have seen, relief often comes at a cost. To knowingly allow someone to suffer without adequate opportunity to benefit from treatments that may reduce their pain is also poor medicine. Good pain management should mean trying to reduce pain as much as possible within the limitations of the side effects and potential for any treatment to be harmful.

If cure and complete relief are not possible, what is the alternative? Is there an approach that offers the ability not just to cope with a life of pain but to enjoy life despite the pain? This book offers just that. To see what this approach is, let's move on to the next part of the book.

'Cure sometimes, relieve often and comfort always...'

Ambroise Paré (c 1510–1590), Royal Surgeon to the Kings of France.

Fact file

- Find a health professional you respect and trust

- Drugs are the most common way of treating pain

- While drugs may be effective, they often only provide partial relief and can have side-effects

- Physical treatments may be helpful for some kinds of pain

- State of mind has a huge impact on our experience of pain and so psychological treatments are helpful

- While treating and relieving pain is the first priority, sometimes a shift to managing pain is needed.

Part two
Finding hope

Chapter 5

Step 1—Relaxation

When it was first suggested that deep, controlled breathing and relaxation could help reduce the pain I was downright angry. Clearly these people had no respect for the agony I was in. However, I agreed to try the approach, the aim being to desensitise the system and 'flick the switch' that confuses pain origin. I was truly amazed. For the first time in my life I felt I had gained some kind of control again over the pain'

Irene, age 55, aged care nurse

Dealing with muscle tension

The place we will start in countering the effects of pain is the body. You may remember that one of the first effects of pain on the body is to switch on and tighten muscles. In other words, the natural response of the muscle to pain is to guard. This is a protective mechanism but over the long term it results in muscle tension which adds to pain and results in changes in posture and the way we move and hold ourselves.

Stress also adds to muscle tension. When we don't adapt well to stress, we react in the way we have been programmed, with the fight or flight response. Any problem (and pain may be a truly severe problem in our lives) can cause our brain to send an alarm signal to the body causing physical changes such as increased heart and breathing rate, increased muscle tension and increased blood pressure.

Hands and feet may get cold as blood is directed to large muscles and away from the digestive system. Our pupils dilate and hearing becomes sharper. If problems are continuous and the stressors of life and of persistent pain seem unrelenting, and we don't learn to deal with them effectively, long-term negative effects to our bodies occur.

Stress is unavoidable and a certain amount of stress is good for us. However, long-term stress from either chronic pain or other circumstances is not good for us and will have other long-term effects on our life. It is important to have ways of dealing with stress and pain that reduce muscle tension and counter these other effects.

Re-energising the body: being relaxed

You will be glad to know that the way to do this and the first skill that we will look at is easy for most people – it is learning to relax. Before we look at how to relax, let's look at how relaxation can help.

Instinctively, we all know that relaxation makes us feel better. Even though we may sometimes find it hard to do, we love getting away to the beach or the bush, watching sport or just sitting under a tree with a good book. Times of relaxation help to refresh us and enable us to face life with renewed energy and enthusiasm. If we don't get enough time to relax, life can become pretty dreary.

Relaxation, however, is more than just avoiding stress. Some types of relaxation have been shown to have beneficial effects on our bodies.

For example, for those who have enjoyed the deeply relaxed feeling that comes from lying in a hot pool or spa, that feeling may come from the release of natural opioids into the body. In fact, the effect can be so powerful that there are reports of some people becoming addicted to it. There is a report in a medical journal of a Japanese woman who bathed regularly in a hot spring to help her skin. However, she could not stop going to the baths several times a day and had to be placed in isolation in hospital for a month to help cure her of her addiction.[1]

Although this may be an extreme case, most of us know that we feel good after relaxing. Not surprisingly, this is backed up by scientific studies that show that relaxation techniques such as deep breathing have very positive effects on the body. These effects include lowering of blood pressure, reduction in muscle tension, slowing of heart rate and improved sleep.

Benefits of relaxation on pain

As well as positive effects on our general health, relaxation has also been shown to have positive effects on pain. People have studied the effects of specific relaxation techniques such as progressive muscle relaxation and found that they reduce stress and muscle tension. Importantly for people with chronic pain though, it does more than relax muscles. It also increases the threshold at which people feel pain. So, when you are relaxed, you feel less pain.

'As well as positive effects on our general health, relaxation has also been shown to have positive effects on pain.'

A number of other studies have been done to look at whether relaxation techniques can reduce pain. These studies have looked at the effect of relaxation in a whole range of pain conditions including arthritis, pain after surgery, headaches and pain related to cancer.[2][3] The good news is that relaxation consistently produces a reduction in pain levels. The type of relaxation technique does not have to be complicated or difficult. Even something as simple as listening to music has been shown to reduce the intensity of pain.[4]

All of this work from scientific studies shows that relaxation is definitely helpful for countering the effects of pain and stress. However, it is not the complete answer. The bulk of evidence suggests that even though relaxation helps reduce pain, the effects are fairly short-lived and although they are useful, relaxation techniques won't eliminate our pain entirely.

Nevertheless, even if they have a fairly short-term effect, relaxation techniques can still be tremendously helpful. They can be used at times when pain and stress levels are high and they can help to reduce stress simply and without side effects. If practised regularly, relaxation also acts to prevent the build-up of pain and stress levels and helps to keep them under a reasonable level of control. Therefore, relaxation is an important first step in learning to overcome pain.

Types of relaxation

There are many ways to relax and you may be wondering whether

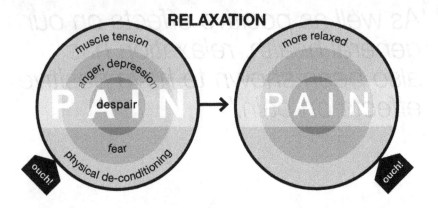

RELAXATION

muscle tension
anger, depression
despair
fear
physical de-conditioning
ouch!

more relaxed
ouch!

one type of relaxation is better than another. In general, the answer is no. The important thing is to find a way of relaxing that you feel comfortable with and that suits you.

The ways in which we relax are countless but basically fall into two types. The first is just doing things that we find relaxing. This includes things like going for a walk, watching television, playing cards, doing crosswords, playing sport, lying on the grass, sleeping, taking a bath, watching the football and going to movies. The second way we relax is by using specific techniques that produce muscle relaxation and a feeling of calm. These include techniques such as deep breathing and muscle relaxation.

Both of these types of relaxation are important and in this chapter we will look at both. First, we will look at what activities you can do to help you to relax. If you don't have one already, it may be very helpful to think through what you can do on a regular basis that makes you feel calmer and more relaxed. Second, we will look at some relaxation techniques. As well as having time for activities in your life that you find relaxing and enjoyable, it is helpful to have a specific technique that counters the effect of pain and stress. If done on a regular basis, this not only helps deal with stress and reduce pain, but can be a preventive strategy that helps prevent the build up of stress, muscle tension and pain.

'It is helpful to have a specific technique that counters the effect of pain and stress.'

Sleep as a relaxation technique

Sleep is one of nature's most important ways of providing our bodies and minds with time out. It is a crucial factor in feeling rested, relaxed and healthy. There are many studies that show that having around seven hours sleep each night is an important factor in staying healthy and feeling good.

We also know that lack of sleep decreases our tolerance and threshold for pain.[5][6] In fact, it has been shown that if you reduce your normal sleep time to four hours, the volume of pain the next day increases by one quarter. In other words, the less sleep, the stronger your pain is likely to be. Of course, all people are different and seven hours is not a magical number. However, it is important that you get as much sleep as you need to function well and minimise your pain.

For many people with chronic pain, this will sound like an impossible task. You may not remember the last time you had a good night's sleep and aiming for seven hours may seem impossible. Although pain does interrupt and interfere with sleep, there are some things you can do to help get a better night's sleep.

As a retired diplomat, I found myself getting overweight, not valuing exercise or sport and developing pain in both hips and knees. I spent every day reading foreign affairs journals, watching political news or engaging in intense discussions with other retired diplomats. I often found myself infuriated when the Foreign Office made 'stupid mistakes'. My doctor warned me that unless I changed my way of life, my pain would increase and my health would suffer further. I became even angrier at first, but eventually took notice of the doctor's advice, began an exercise and weight loss program, and most importantly learned a simple relaxation technique. Relaxation was only part of the answer, but as I began this new approach, relaxation helped me plan and live a healthier life. In several months my pain decreased and I'm glad to be enjoying this new way of life.

Richard, age 68, retired diplomat

Tips for a better night's sleep

Simple skills may help to maximise the length and quality of your sleep. For example:

○ Going to bed at a regular time each day. This helps your body clock to become tuned.

○ Having a regular bedtime routine or activity such as reading or listening to calming music. This also helps your mind to switch into sleep mode.

○ Avoid becoming dependent on sleeping tablets or alcohol. Even though it is tempting when you are lying there watching the ceiling, medications are not a good way to solve the problem.

'Going to bed at a regular time each day. This helps your body clock to become tuned.'

○ Getting some time outside during the day. If you exercise at the same time, it is even better. Both exercise and being outside help the body to produce chemicals that make it easier for us to sleep more easily and deeply.

○ Making sure that your analgesia is optimal. This does not mean having enough analgesia so that your pain is gone and you can get to sleep. But it does mean that if you are taking medications for your pain that you take them at the right time to reduce your pain for as much of the night as possible.

○ Avoid things that decrease your chance of sleeping well such as lots of coffee or caffeinated soft drinks, especially before going to bed.

○ Avoid long naps or dozing during the late afternoon or evening. If for some reason you feel very tired during the day, take a short nap but do it early in the afternoon and limit it to 30 to 60 minutes.

○ Anything more than this will further disrupt your sleep cycle and make it harder to rest well at night.

Relaxing activities

As we said earlier, we can either relax by doing things we naturally enjoy and find calming or we can use specific relaxation techniques. Let us look first at activities that help us relax.

'Doing what we find relaxing sounds as though it should be easy but pain or busyness can make it much harder...'

Doing what we find relaxing sounds as though it should be easy but pain or busyness can make it much harder than it sounds. Hobbies and sports that people used to enjoy can become difficult or even impossible to do because of pain. When people can't do them anymore, they lose out on regular exercise, fun and interaction with friends. This makes them even more out of condition and depressed.

To stop this cycle, it is very important to find something you can do on a regular basis that provides you with enjoyment and that helps you to feel relaxed. Even though you may not be able to do what you used to enjoy, try to think of something you can still do that you would find relaxing.

Here are some examples of relaxing activities that you can do, although of course there are many more. Use this as a starting point to think about something you could do on a regular basis that would give you some times of relaxation.

Relaxing activities

Taking a nap

Going for a walk

Watching a comedy

Listening to music

Watching TV

Aromatherapy

Doing a crossword

Hypnosis

Having a massage

Closing your eyes and daydreaming

Playing with your pet

Playing with your children

Reading a book

Reading the paper

Making a quilt

Going sailing

Sitting quietly

Woodworking

Origami

Painting or drawing

Cooking

Sitting in a hot spa

Lying down on the grass and closing your eyes

Doing a jigsaw puzzle

Taking a bath

Doing tai chi

Going fishing

'Many of these relaxation techniques are based around breathing or muscle relaxation or a combination of these approaches.'

Relaxation techniques

While doing something relaxing on a regular basis is important for our physical and mental health, there are a number of relaxation techniques can also reduce muscle tension and stress. Many of these relaxation techniques are based around breathing or muscle relaxation or a combination of these approaches. They can be used on a regular basis to help keep our pain and tension levels to a minimum. They can also be used to reduce pain in situations where we are experiencing increased pain or stress. For example, many people find a simple breathing technique helpful for facing a stressful situation such as going to the dentist or having to talk in public. You can use it beforehand to increase your sense of calm and control over the situation.

Described below are several techniques based on breathing and muscle relaxation that are widely used and that have been shown to have positive effects on pain and muscle tension. The important thing is to find one that suits you and your lifestyle and that you can easily put into practice on a regular basis. You may like to try these different techniques and find one that you are comfortable with and that seems to work for you. You may also like to explore others that you can find on the internet or in other books.

Becoming more flexible

I'd had a passion for fine industrial tools in high school, decided on tool-making as a career, and always loved my work. But there was an unfortunate catch - after years of leaning over the workbench, focussing closely on hand-finishing precision tools I found my upper back had become chronically stiff and painful. I entered a pain program and found great benefit from becoming aware of my posture and beginning to become aware of my body through an exercise in body awareness. Not only did I benefit from focussing daily on a body awareness protocol, I also found my pain decreased as I remembered to straighten my upper back rather than remain hunched over my workbench. As I did this I became more flexible and when that happened, to my surprise, my mind also became more flexible and I became more my old self. I had become an angry person, at least partly because of my pain.

Harry, age 57, tool-maker

Breathing techniques

Breathing is such a natural part of our lives that we don't pay much attention to the breath itself. And sometimes we become so involved in what we are doing that we forget to breathe properly!

When we become stressed, anxious or in pain our breathing becomes shallow, and we fail to supply enough oxygen to our bodies, and to our brains! Breathing well is the basis of the relaxation techniques that we suggest you use as part of your everyday routine.

To focus your attention on breathing, begin to practice this exercise daily:

○ Bring your attention to the rise and fall of your abdomen as you breathe. Gently place your hands on your abdomen and follow your breathing.

○ Is your chest moving in harmony with your abdomen or is it rigid? Allow your chest to follow your abdomen.

○ Now try some deep breaths. You may be lying down or seated.

○ Inhale slowly and deeply through your nose and exhale through your mouth. Your mouth, jaw, and tongue will be relaxed. Take long, slow, deep breaths that raise and lower your abdomen. Focus on the sound and feeling of breathing as you become more and more relaxed.

○ Continue deep breathing for about five or ten minutes at a time, once or twice a day for a week or two. Then, if you like, extend the period to twenty minutes.

Body awareness

Many of us can become so occupied with what we are doing during the day that our minds become caught up with thoughts of pain and with the problems that pain seems to bring with it. Focusing on the body with awareness is a strategy that we can use to help calm and relax the mind. It is easy to do, and you will be able to do it with your eyes open or closed.

We simply focus on each part of the body, starting with the feet. Here is how:

○ First focus on your feet, noticing the sensation of the soles of your feet against your socks or shoes.

○ Next, move to the calves of your legs, perhaps noticing the feeling of your trousers against your legs, then your thighs, and if you are seated notice the sensation of your thighs pressing against the chair; then your buttocks and pelvic area, noting any tension in that area; move now to your back, noticing your spine and the clothing on your back; move to the chest and abdomen, noticing the movement of this area as you breathe.

○ Now become aware of your hands, lower arms and upper arms. Move now to your neck and shoulders; pay particular attention to this area of your body, as we often become tense in the neck and shoulders.

○ Finally move to your face, forehead, eyes, nose, cheeks, mouth, then ears and scalp. Pause now and become aware of your whole body in space. This takes only a few minutes of your time, and you can do it anywhere, several times each day!

Whole body tension/relaxation

This relaxation technique is a fairly simple muscle relaxation technique that does not focus on one muscle group but simply aims to produce generalised relaxation through the body. Here's how it's done:

○ Tense everything in your whole body; stay with that tension.

○ Hold it as long as you can without feeling pain.

○ Slowly release the tension and very gradually feel it leave your body.

○ Repeat three times.

Progressive muscle relaxation

Progressive muscle relaxation builds on good breathing and can be practised lying down or sitting in a chair. Our aim is to achieve deep muscle relaxation:

○ We begin by tensing each muscle group for five to seven seconds, and then relaxing that same group for about 10 seconds. You may wish to tighten and relax each group twice.

○ Curl both fists, tightening upper and lower arms, hold, and then relax.

○ Wrinkle the muscles in your face as if you were a small child poking faces at your playmate, hold, then relax.

○ Tighten the muscles of the neck and shoulders, hold, and then relax.

○ Tighten the chest and upper back, hold, and then relax.

○ Tighten the lower abdomen, low back, buttocks and pelvic area, hold, and then relax.

○ Tighten the thighs, hold, and then relax.

○ Tighten the lower legs, hold, and then relax.

○ Curl the feet and toes as if into a ball, hold, then relax.

Meditation techniques

Meditation techniques are a popular way of relaxing and dealing with stress. These can be very effective in helping us physically, but they rely more strongly on engaging the mind than the other breathing and muscle relaxation techniques. We will explore meditation techniques further when we look at using the mind to overcome pain.

Relaxation—making it part of your life

It is important to consider how to make relaxation a part of your life. As mentioned earlier, this book outlines some simple skills that will increase your ability to control your pain. However, to be effective and to enable you to do this, they must become part of your life and they can do so only if you put them into action.

At the end of each of the next five chapters, you will find a section like this that encourages and challenges you to think of what steps you are going to take to put these skills into place. Some of these may not be possible to do immediately. However, it may be helpful to have a firm commitment written into your daily schedule or written on your calendar. It may also be useful to talk over your plan with someone else. This helps to make sure that you are not taking on too much and helps you to follow through.

Decide what you will do to relax

○ Consider what **activities** you can do to relax. Think about activities that you enjoy and that you think would be fun and relaxing but suit your body, your limitations and your lifestyle. If you haven't done them before but they sound enjoyable and feasible, you may like to experiment. Of course, you can always change in the future and you may like to have several, but choose at least one activity that you can do on a regular basis that will help you to relax.

○ Choose a relaxation **technique** that suits you. Start with the ones described in this book but feel free to explore others. Find a technique that you feel comfortable with and that can be done simply and easily as part of your schedule.

Decide when you are going to relax

○ Relaxing activities may be regular or semi-regular events, depending on what they are. A relaxation technique, on the other hand, should be more frequent and regular and ideally should be done several times a week. If you are relaxing on a regular basis, five to 10 minutes a day may be enough. Alternatively, you may like to get a slightly longer time several times a week.

○ The time of day does not matter, although some people find that the evening is a good time. This allows you to deal with the tensions and stresses of the day. It also helps your body to prepare for sleep. Relaxation can maximise the good that we obtain from sleep, by preparing our bodies and deepening sleep.

○ As a suggestion, try and set apart five to 10 minutes toward the end of the day to quieten, relax and let go of stress and tension. No matter how good you may feel, make a commitment to yourself to set aside this time at least three times a week and make relaxation part of your life.

○ Although some people prefer the evening to relax, this may be difficult or impractical for several reasons. If it is difficult, try to find another time during the day when it is easier to get in a few minutes of uninterrupted relaxation.

○ As well as a regular time of relaxation, you may like to use other opportunities to practice your technique and relax. For example, if you catch public transport, you may be able to use this time to practise your favourite relaxation technique. You may like to take some time out during a lunch break to sit in a park and relax. Or take a few minutes to relax when the children are having a nap.

These little times can be important fuse breakers that help to reduce stress, tension and pain and keep you relaxed and calm.

Decide where you are going to relax

○ As well as finding a time, it is also important to find a place for your relaxation technique. If you can, find somewhere that can be your quiet place. It may be a comfortable chair, it may be under a tree, beside a lake, or in the backyard. This is your place, a place to retreat to when you feel the need to relax or deal with your pain. It is preferable then to find a place where you know you won't be distracted and can practice relaxation without wondering if you will be disturbed. Remember though, it is important not to make this the only place you can relax! Vary the place from time to time so that you learn to relax almost anywhere.

○ Being undisturbed may not be easy. It may require you to take the phone off the hook or turn off your mobile. It may also require help from others. If you have two or three young children, it is often next to impossible to find a space in the day that is truly uninterrupted. If this is the case, ask your partner or a friend to take over and to give you some time when you know you are not going to have to deal with anything else.

Have a plan to maintain this new skill

It is said that it takes 66 days to build a habit. Even though being more relaxed may not sound that hard, making it part of our lives as a regular habit is not always easy.

Habits are helped by committing to a regular time over a certain period and maybe checking in with someone to make sure it is done. To help maintain your commitment, you may like to:

○ Write down a plan for when you are going to relax and tick it off when it is done.

○ Be accountable—get a friend to check how you are going on a semi-regular basis.

○ Mix it up. Relaxing in the same way all the time will almost certainly get boring. Try different activities and techniques and change them from time to time.

Summing up

Relaxation is good for us. It helps counteract the effect of stress and
pain in our lives. It not only lessens pain but also reduces muscle
tension and makes us feel better. Take some time out now to work
out how you are going to build relaxation into your life.

Fact file: Relaxation

- Pain is a stressor.

- Stress creates physical tension.

- Tension adds to pain.

- Relaxation reduces the effects of stress.

- Relaxation helps relieve pain.

- We can relax by using specific relaxation techniques.

- We can relax by doing other activities that we find enjoyable.

Chapter 6

Step 2—Exercise

I live with arthritis in my spine. On some days the pain is hard to manage even with medication. If I didn't do my walk and a few exercises in the morning, I would be confined to a chair.

Denise, age 78, mother of 3, grandmother to 8

Rebuilding the body: being active

People with chronic pain can get caught in a cycle where they avoid activity because it makes the pain worse. This results in physical deconditioning that contributes further to pain. The big question is: how can we break out of this cycle and reverse the deconditioning? How can we make our bodies stronger and at the same time reduce our pain?

The answer of course will come as no surprise. We know that being active helps to strengthen muscles and increases blood flow to all parts of the body. When we are fit, we feel better and can do things more easily.

In the last chapter, we looked at relaxation as the first step in rebuilding our bodies so that we can face pain and find hope. Exercising and being active is a balance to relaxation. Both being relaxed and being active complement each other and work together to get us in the best possible physical shape.

If you have chronic pain though, it is almost certain that you have a problem that is running through your mind. You probably would like to be more active but you have tried and it just makes your pain worse. Being more active may seem impossible.

We know that this is a big issue for people with pain and in fact it is such a big issue that we will address it twice; once in this chapter, and again in a following chapter. We will give you some skills that help get past this so that you can become active and enjoy the benefits that it can bring. Before we do that though, let's look at some of the good things that being active will do for us.

The general benefits of being active

There is no doubt that being active is good for us. The first and most obvious benefit of being active is that it makes us stronger.

However, it has been shown to be helpful in other ways. Being active:

○ Helps maintain a healthy blood pressure and improves heart function.

○ Has positive effects on our immune system that helps fight disease.

○ Can help reduce weight. This is not only good for our general health but decreases pain by reducing the load on our muscles, ligaments and joints.

○ Helps our minds as well as our bodies. Being active results in the release of chemicals that improve our mood and make us feel better. It is not surprising then that scientific studies show that many forms of exercise have positive effects on anger and depression.

○ Helps us sleep better. The chemicals that improve mood also help us sleep well. In turn, improved sleep further reduces anxiety and tension, improves mood and relieves pain.

○ Increases our brain power. Particularly in older people, it has been shown that regular activity not only makes people feel better but also improves mental performance.[1]

In summary, being active benefits fitness and health and improves sleep, mood and mental performance.

The benefits of being active for pain

Being active has many benefits for the mind and body, but does it help pain? The good news is, yes! Scientists have shown that being active helps with pain[2] [3] and also releases beneficial chemicals that relieve pain.[4] As an example, the naturally occurring (or endogenous) feel-good chemicals are opioids like morphine and other strong painkillers. You may have heard of runner's high. This is the state of wellbeing that runners feel when they have been jogging for some time. This high is caused by the release of these natural opioids.

These chemicals also result in pain relief. Careful measurements during scientific studies have shown that, immediately following exercise, our pain threshold—the level at which something feels

EXERCISE

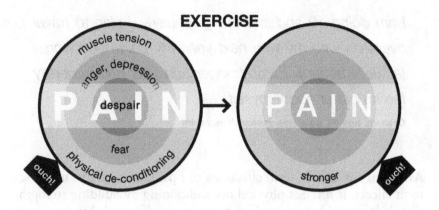

painful—is much higher. So we feel less pain. This is one reason why people can often have quite serious injuries while playing sport and yet seem to be unaware of any pain.

Ouch—that hurts! The physiotherapist at the pain clinic told me I had to start moving because my muscles were losing strength. I said to myself you must be joking—it hurts me to move—better to be deconditioned than put myself through more pain and need to take more painkillers! I had become so fearful of moving—a prisoner in my own home. I started with one or two exercises three times a day. The physio told me that people who have had pain for a long time usually take longer to recover from exercise initially due to the effects of new loading patterns on muscles. It took me a long while to believe her—but she was right. The pain in my hips and back did get better over time as my muscles got stronger. I set goals for the first time in 10 years. Success builds on success! I started with two exercises a day and now

I am doing 10 and swimming regularly. I plan to travel overseas with my wife next year. My pain is no worse (actually better!). I am stronger and fitter and generally feeling better about myself.

Graham, age 48, amputee, research assistant

As well as these short term effects on our pain, being active has long-term effects. It reverses physical deconditioning by building strength. This helps provide increased support for our bones, helps to correct postural problems and makes pain less likely when we exercise next time.

What type of exercise works best?

You may be keen to get these benefits from being active but wondering if some types of activity are better than others. The short answer is yes. Strenuous activity is more likely to result in the release of feel-good chemicals such as endogenous opioids. Activity must be fairly high in intensity (certainly enough to make you out of breath) to release these feel-good chemicals.

If the thought of doing vigorous exercise sounds daunting, here is some good news—it only has to be short. In fact, it has been shown that three minutes of vigorous exercise is enough to get endogenous opioid release. This compares with even very long sessions of light exercise which will do very little to trigger release of opioids.

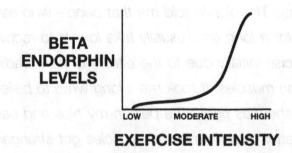

'Although vigorous activity gives strong benefits by the release of endogenous opioids, you can still get significant benefits from light exercise.'

This doesn't mean that light exercise is a waste of time. But it does mean that if you can push yourself to the point where the exercise is strenuous, you get the additional benefits of the release of those natural opioids. Like opioids that come in bottles, packets and syringes, these chemicals improve our mood, make us feel relaxed and reduce pain – good reasons to try to get to a level where our exercise is vigorous!

But I can't do that!

Some of you may be feeling despondent at this point. You are keen to get the benefits of being more active and would like to be able to reduce your pain by releasing these chemicals. But doing vigorous exercise is just not an option.

The good news is that although vigorous activity gives strong benefits by the release of endogenous opioids, you can still get significant benefits from light exercise. These benefits come through other means that also result in improvements in the body as well as mood. Even mild exercise such as a gentle form of yoga has been shown to produce a reduction in muscle tension as well as a reduction in anger and depression.[5] Regular light exercise for as little as five minutes a day or 15 minutes three times a week has also been shown to reduce pain in people with low back problems.

You don't have to get to the point of being out of breath or in pain to get the benefits. No matter how little you can do, regular exercise will help.

When activity makes your pain worse

For some people with chronic pain, even light exercise may seem impossible. In these situations, it is helpful to work out why exercise is not possible. Are you worried about causing further damage? Perhaps any activity causes so much pain that it feels impossible. Or it may not cause pain immediately but you have learned from experience that you will suffer later.

These are all powerful reasons for avoiding exercise and it is important to address them. We will deal further with fear of damage in a later chapter. However, if you do feel that way it may be important to consult with your health professional. Check with them that it is safe for you to exercise and ask whether there are activities that you need to avoid. Being active may still hurt, but remember that pain does not necessarily mean you are causing damage! This is such an important message that we will come back to it later.

Increasing your activity levels

Once you are confident that you are not causing damage, there are two simple steps to increasing what you can do and minimising your pain. The first step is a very basic concept called pacing, which is used in many pain management programs. Simply break up your activities into manageable portions so that they don't result in a flare-up of pain. So when you try to increase your activity levels, break them into portions, no matter how good you feel or how determined you are to get the job done. Even on a good day don't try to mow the whole lawn or vacuum the whole house! No matter how tempted you are, don't! Break the task into manageable chunks that won't cause a huge increase in pain.

The second step is to pace upwards. Once you have decided what is a reasonable chunk of activity, work out a plan for gradually increasing it. As you increase your activity levels, take them slowly and plan for adequate times of rest and relaxation as you build up your strength and exercise tolerance levels. Work out an activity program that is manageable for where you are at the moment. Even setting something that is below what you feel you can accomplish will work. The important thing is to plan small increasing steps in how much you do.

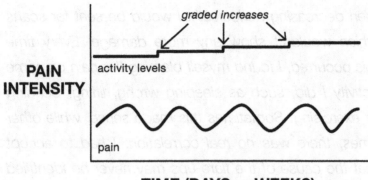

PAIN INTENSITY

graded increases

activity levels

pain

TIME (DAYS or WEEKS)

For example, it may be difficult for you to walk 50 metres without being in severe pain. If that is the case, plan to walk 40 metres or even 25 metres for the first week. Each week increase this by 10 per cent (two and a half metres).

Although this may seem a small amount, if you start with 25 metres and increase the amount you walk by 10 per cent each week, by three months you will be walking 80 metres, by six months you will be walking 270 metres and, if you keep this up, by 12 months you will be walking three kilometres!

I've had lower back pain with associated leg pain for 25 years and have had to endure countless flare-ups of this pain over the years. This has caused me huge anxiety and makes planning for future events very stressful. It's the seemingly unexplainable flare-ups which puzzle me. I can do the same thing every day of my life and suffer pain one day and no pain the next. I have asked my doctor why I continue to get flare-ups and most of the time, no good answer is provided. It can be extremely frustrating. My sciatic pain would just keep increasing then decreasing periodically. I would be sent for scans which wouldn't show any more damage. Every time this occurred, I found myself blaming the pain on some activity I did, such as sleeping wrong, lifting, bending or exercising. Sometimes this made sense, while other times, there was no real correlation. I had to accept that the cause of the flare-ups may never be identified and they are part of the natural cycle when you have chronic pain.

Judith, age 70, retired teacher

Dealing with flare-ups

In Chapter 2, How Does Pain Work? we talked about flare-ups. These are the times when pain temporarily increases due to various factors. Regular exercise is one of the best ways to reduce the frequency and intensity of flare-ups. It is helpful to be able to deal with them effectively so they are not as severe and don't last as long. Here are some tips for dealing with flare-ups:

○ Decide if the increase in pain is a flare-up, rather than a new pain. A flare-up will be pain in the same place and will be the same type of pain as usual, but more severe. If it is the same type of pain, it is unlikely that you need to see your doctor. However, if you have new symptoms of illness such as fever, vomiting, or numbness, these should be reported.

○ Remember that a flare-up does not necessarily mean more damage. It is the body responding to a change in posture, movement, activity or other factors that increase pain and it will settle with time.

○ Identify if you have been overdoing things physically or are tired or stressed in any way. If you are doing too much, you may need to pace or alter your activities.

○ Use relaxation skills to help counter the pain and reduce stress.

'Stretching is an extremely valuable skill in treating chronic pain. If you have pain, it is almost certain that surrounding muscles have tightened as a natural reaction to protect the body.'

○ In the first two to three days, techniques such as application of heat may help reduce the pain.

○ Don't stop everything. It may help to reduce activity by 25 to 50 per cent for several days, but keep doing some exercise and make a plan to gradually increase to your previous exercise routine.

○ Continue to use your medication as prescribed and try to avoid jumping to a higher dose. If it is essential, see it as a temporary measure and aim to return to your normal dose as soon as possible.

Stretching

Stretching is a form of physical exercise in which a specific muscle or group of muscles is deliberately stretched. In its most basic form, stretching is a natural and instinctive activity; it is performed by humans and many animals. For example, when we get a cramp at night, the instinctive response is to get up and stretch it out to relieve the pain. And how many times does a cat stretch each day, particularly after sleeping!

Regular stretching decreases stiffness, increases flexibility and increases movement in our joints.

Stretching is an extremely valuable skill in treating chronic pain. If you have pain, it is almost certain that surrounding muscles have tightened as a natural reaction to protect the body. Muscles that are tight can limit movement of joints and eventually cause long term postural problems. Changes in posture and limitations in movement can often make pain worse.

A regular, whole body stretching program helps to reverse these changes. Stretching lengthens muscles that have become tight. This decreases stiffness, increases flexibility and corrects postural changes, helping you to move more freely.

For all these reasons, it is very important to include stretching as a regular part of your daily schedule. This is even more vital if you spend long sessions in the same position such as sitting at a desk and using a computer or if pain makes it difficult to maintain your normal posture.

Stretches can be done in a number of ways that suit your lifestyle. Before doing any sort of exercise, it is helpful to do some stretching. It is also helpful to take a few minutes to stretch if you have been sitting for some length of time. We would recommend that any time you spend an hour sitting, take three to five minutes each hour to stretch. Doing this is helpful in preventing muscle tension and pain developing.

Whatever your lifestyle, stretching is important in reversing the changes caused by pain. To help, we have provided a set of stretching exercises at the back of this book. These exercises stretch many of the muscles that are affected in people with chronic pain. To learn about stretching you may also like to consult your physiotherapist. They will be able to work with you to find a set of stretching exercises that suit you and the sort of pain you have. They are not difficult and with a little practice can become a beneficial part of your daily routine.

Strength training

What is strength training?

As well as activities that build general fitness, it is useful to do activities that build strength. Strength training is also known as resistance training or weight lifting. These exercises are designed to increase the power of the muscles. Strong muscles help to support and take pressure off painful joints. Strengthening exercises can also have a good effect on bones and have been shown to reduce the number of falls in older people.

'The encouraging news is that it has been shown that older people who may feel out of condition but exercise are still able to regain muscle strength and bulk.'

What happens to our muscles as we get older?

In general, as we grow, our muscles get bigger until early adulthood. But then, with normal ageing and a relatively inactive lifestyle, most people lose 20 to 40 per cent of their muscle mass by the age of 80. Muscle fibres shrink and are replaced by fat and connective tissue. Muscle fibres then become harder to stimulate and less able to produce the energy needed to do activities without getting tired. The amount of fuel (food) that your muscles can store becomes less, and their ability to take oxygen from the bloodstream is reduced.

The result of all these changes is that as we get older our muscles become smaller and weaker, and get tired more quickly than when we were young. It is not known why all these changes happen, but it is clear that many of these changes probably have more to do with decreased physical activity levels rather than the normal ageing process. The encouraging news is that it has been shown that older people who may feel out of condition but exercise are still able to regain muscle strength and bulk.

How will I benefit from strength training?

Strength training will make your muscles stronger. So anything that requires muscle strength, such as getting out of a chair, climbing stairs or carrying shopping will become much easier.

Strength training can also increase your metabolism, so it can help you lose body fat, particularly if you also lower your intake of calories.

As well as these changes to your muscles, strength training also makes the ligaments that attach to bones and the bones themselves stronger, reducing the chance of future injury and osteoporotic fractures.

Chronic pain or any condition that decreases mobility and leads to muscle shrinkage will benefit from strength training. Over time you will find that, as your muscle strength improves, your ability to perform the normal activities of daily life improves—the simple task of getting out of a chair, for example, doesn't take as much energy to perform.

Ways to be active

Walking

Walking is a simple way of being active that is possible for most people. You can start at any level and work up. It is not harmful to your joints, can be done nearly anywhere, can be enjoyed with a friend and is known to be beneficial. If you have not walked a long distance for some time, you should check with your health professional first. Then, when you have the all clear, start slowly. Choose a distance you think is manageable, no matter how small. Then, increase the length and pace of your walk gradually. Here are some tips on how to get started and how to prepare for walking:

○ Wear comfortable and lightweight shoes with good support.

○ Do a few warm-up exercises and stretches first.

○ Walk at a steady pace and stand as straight as you can.

○ Start with a five-minute walk and then increase gradually. Aim to increase the length of time to 30 minutes. Try to walk at least three times per week.

Other ways to exercise

If walking is not possible, there are many other types of exercise that you may like to consider. For example you may like aquarobics, Tai Chi, yoga, wheelchair basketball, dancing or swimming. Ideally choose an activity that suits you and your abilities. Find one or two that you can do regularly without too much trouble, that you enjoy and that help to maintain and build your physical fitness levels.

Exercise—Making it part of your life

What can I do to exercise and become more active?

Decide on an activity

○ You may like to walk but if walking does not suit you or you are unable to walk, choose another activity. It is quite possible, particularly when you start, that it may increase the pain. But if it is something that you normally enjoy, it is going to be easier to do and maintain.

○ Find an activity that is relatively simple to start and do. It is better if it does not require a lot of equipment, expense or preparation. The simpler it is, the more likely you are to do it and keep doing it over the long term.

○ Find an activity level that you can manage. If you can, try to get some vigorous exercise, even in small bursts. If you can't, remember that even light exercise is helpful and stick with that.

○ Explore types of exercise that minimise the strain on the area where you get pain. For example, for people with low back pain, water activities such as aquarobics and deep-water running can allow them to engage in vigorous exercise with less impact on the spine.

Have a plan to increase

Once you have chosen what you are going to do, work out how you are going to increase what you can do to gradually build condition. It does not matter what type of exercise you do as long as you do it regularly and for a decent length of time. Have a goal and work toward it.

○ Most health experts agree that regular, moderate intensity exercise for at least 30 minutes around three to five times a week is beneficial. This 30 minutes doesn't have to be done in one go but can be broken into smaller sessions.

○ If you are not getting this much exercise already, plan to build it into your day. It is always best to start small and build up. Build up using either a time measure or another measure that suits the activity such as measuring the distance you walk.

○ If you use a time measure, you could consider the following schedule. Start with one five minute session a day. Continue that for one month and then increase this to 10 minutes. Each month add another five minutes to your exercise routine. Aim to spend at least 30 minutes each day being active.

○ If you walk and want to measure distance, you may like to use a pedometer. Start at a reasonable distance that you can achieve without too much pain. Then gradually increase the distance you walk each week. For example, increase by 10 per cent each week.

Have a plan to maintain this new skill

It is one thing to reach your goal but it is sometimes difficult to maintain. Here are some hints that may make it easier to maintain over the long term so that you can continue to enjoy the benefits that being active will bring.

○ Ask someone to join you. Many people find it useful to exercise with a friend. Find someone you like being with and who enjoys the same type of exercise as you at the pace you feel comfortable with. This will make it more enjoyable and easier to stick to a regular time of exercise.

○ Join a group. Team sports and group physical activity programs can also be good for a similar reason. Organised activities can be an opportunity to get out and meet people. Being active with the right group of people can be a lot more fun than just doing exercise alone. And the more enjoyable it is, the more likely you are to stick at it over the long term.

○ Mix it up. Doing the same activity all the time can get boring. Mix up what you do and change the activity from time to time or do it in a different place or different way. This will help keep it interesting and enjoyable.

Summing up

Exercising is good for us! It helps counteract the effect of stress and pain in our lives and promotes physical and mental strength. No matter what we are facing, being active on a regular basis helps us face pain and live happier and healthier lives. Take some time now to work out how to make being active a regular part of your life.

Fact file: Exercise

- Pain results in physical deconditioning.

- Physical deconditioning adds to pain.

- Being active has general health benefits.

- Being active helps relieve pain.

- We can be active by engaging in a graduated walking program.

- We can be active by engaging in other activities that we enjoy.

Chapter 7

Step 3—Gratitude

I love to go out on the balcony at night and look at the sky and the clouds and trees. I learnt to gradually remember some of the day's events and steps I had taken for which I could honestly be grateful.

Pat, age 72, teacher

Rebuilding the mind: changing the way we think

There is an old saying that a sound body will lead to a sound mind. So far in the book, we have focused on the physical—the re-energising and rebuilding of our bodies. As we have seen, there is now a lot of evidence that shows that both being relaxed and being active make us physically stronger and healthier people.

As well, there is much we can do that makes us stronger mentally which also helps overcome our pain. The next two chapters will focus on two attitudes that counter the effects of pain on the mind: gratitude and courage. Both of them are hugely important and not only make us feel better, they can also help deal with pain.

Pain and acceptance

Before looking at gratitude, let us first touch on another way of thinking that is now widely regarded as being important in dealing with pain: acceptance. There is much evidence that building acceptance is very helpful in dealing not only with the physical aspects of pain, but also the emotions associated with it such as depression and anger.

Many people don't like the idea of acceptance because it seems passive—it suggests giving in to the fact that they will always have pain. If you have pain, who wants to be told that you have to stop looking to get better and just accept the fact that you are going to have pain for the rest of your life? No wonder acceptance has an image problem!

To further explore acceptance, it may be helpful to look at what it is and what it isn't. First, acceptance isn't passive. It is not meekly accepting that you will always have pain and that there is nothing you can do about it. Second, acceptance is not giving up.

It is not saying that this is as good as it gets and that my pain (or my life) will never get any better.

Acceptance is active rather than passive. It is a conscious decision to think and act in a certain way in the face of pain, to live with the hope that life will be better, while acknowledging that the way forward may be different.

This anonymous poem expresses the importance of acceptance:

This is how it is.

Not how it

- was

- might have been

- should have been

Not how I

- wanted it to be

- hoped it would be

- planned it would be

I accept that this is how it is.

Now I will get on with my life the best way I can.

'Acceptance is active rather than passive. It is a conscious decision to think and act in a certain way in the face of pain...'

Acceptance: the way forward

Understandably, the person in pain wants to reclaim the life they used to enjoy. And obviously the obstacle to getting that life back again is the pain. All efforts then are focused on getting rid of it.

The problem with this focus is that it may not be possible, or at least, not possible right now. Pinning all of our hopes on reclaiming a previous quality of life in the face of an immovable obstacle is a recipe for even more frustration, anger, and depression. As long as our happiness is dependent on the pain going away, it will be impossible to enjoy life in the presence of pain.

Acceptance offers another way forward. It is still living with the possibility and hope that pain may go away. However, it is acknowledging that the pain is there and at the moment shows no sign of disappearing. It is acknowledging that it has changed the way you feel and think about life. And it is acknowledging that pain has changed your ability to do many of the things that you used to love.

Acceptance does not mean that we just sit there and mourn what has been lost.

It took me years to accept that this pain is not going to go away and it is something I am going to have to live with.

Josh, age 25, garden landscaper

The benefits of acceptance

There is no doubt that acceptance ultimately brings a greater peace. Much of the work that tells us about the benefits of acceptance comes from studies of people with cancer. People who have a hard time accepting their diagnosis of cancer struggle with feelings of depression and anger and some even die without truly accepting it.

On the other hand, people who accept their diagnosis deal with it better. They are able to move forward. Many people in the last months of their life find hope and pleasure in life by enjoying even more the things they still have.

Research shows the same trend with people who have other problems, such as chronic pain. People who accept it feel better and are more active. The evidence for the benefits of acceptance is so strong that many pain management centres and programs now include acceptance-based treatments as part of their program. At the same time as trying to provide the best relief possible, they also work with people to help build acceptance and move forward.

Pain and gratitude: you've got to be joking!

Having looked at acceptance, let us now explore the power of gratitude. In doing so, we are heading into new and challenging territory. We could very easily be misunderstood. Some people may have already reacted to the idea of gratitude as ridiculous or impossible. For some with pain, the sadness and anger are so overwhelming that the thought of being thankful is just too silly to think about.

It is important to make clear at the beginning that we are not suggesting that turning from anger, pain and sadness to gratitude is easy. However, many people, even in the most traumatic of situations, have shown that it is possible. And very much like the physical skills, no matter how hard they seem at the beginning, with practice they become easier to use.

So gratitude may sound like a strange thing to be talking about in a book about pain. If you have pain, it is very easy to think there is not much to be thankful about. But there is now increasing scientific evidence that shows the benefits of gratitude.

'If you have pain, it is very easy to think there is not much to be thankful about. But there is now increasing scientific evidence that shows the benefits of gratitude.'

What science tells us about gratitude

A number of studies have now been done to examine how gratitude affects us. In one study, a group of university students were divided into three groups and asked to keep a diary of their feelings as well as their physical symptoms and behaviour over 10 weeks. One group was asked to record up to five major events that affected them during the week, a second group was asked to record five minor hassles and the third group was asked to record five things for which they were thankful. The thankful group did much better than the other two groups. When compared to the group that focused on their hassles, they reported fewer physical symptoms, spent more time being active, were more optimistic and felt better about their lives as a whole.

This study is similar to a number of other studies that show two things. One is that gratitude is good for you. It is definitely linked to feeling better and doing more. The second is that gratitude, as a way of thinking, can be learnt. The students in the group that did better were not chosen because they were naturally more optimistic or thankful or happier. They were all chosen randomly and at the beginning had very similar happiness levels. Doing a simple mental exercise just once a week was enough to change the way they felt about themselves and their circumstances.

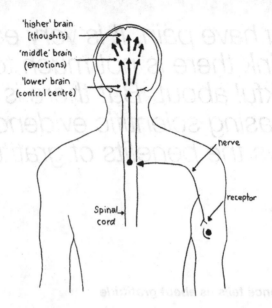

'higher' brain (thoughts)

'middle' brain (emotions)

'lower' brain (control centre)

nerve

receptor

Spinal cord

How does gratitude help our pain?

To look at how gratitude helps our pain, it is helpful to look again at how our body works.

In the early chapters, we described how pain travels from the part of the body that is hurt into the spinal cord and up to the brain. We will now spend a little more time looking at what happens when it reaches the brain. Not only is it fascinating, but as you will also see, it is hugely important for pain management.

We have already described how pain reaches the base of the brain and triggers automatic reactions such as increasing our blood pressure and heart rate. We also described how as the pain messages go higher in the brain, they trigger more complicated emotions like fear or anger. What we didn't talk much about was the final step in our perception of pain: our thoughts. Our thoughts are what give voice to our experience of pain, even if that voice is in our own heads and not spoken aloud

Our thoughts in response to pain can vary enormously. However, the natural way that we respond to pain is negative. Typically we respond with thoughts such as: 'I am sick of this pain', 'I wonder if I have done more damage?' or 'Is this ever going to go away?'.

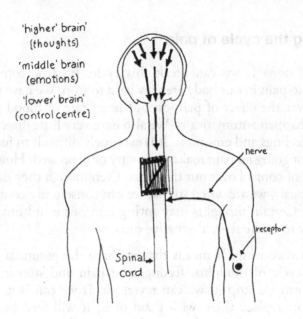

'higher' brain
(thoughts)

'middle' brain
(emotions)

'lower' brain
(control centre)

nerve

receptor

Spinal
cord

Our thoughts affect our pain

What now happens is the most important part of understanding how our thoughts and pain are linked. The processes in our brain do not stop with our thoughts, but respond back down the same pathway. Negative thoughts produce negative feelings and these feelings then feed back into the base of the brain—the control centre for blood pressure, heart rate and other basic body functions. Again, negative feelings will have negative effects on how our body functions.

It is this control centre at the base of the brain that is vitally important in experiencing pain. This area of the brain has direct connections down the spinal cord to the 'gates' that are controlling the amount of pain coming up to the brain. Negative feelings act on the command centre to open the gate and positive feelings act on the command centre to close the gate.

This means that because of this pathway in the brain and spinal cord from our thoughts to our feelings to the control centre for the gates, there are strong links between our thoughts and our pain. Not only does pain go up to the brain to trigger negative responses in our body, feelings and thoughts. Negative thoughts also come back down again to trigger more bad feelings, more negative responses in our body and more pain.

Breaking the cycle of pain

The good news is we can break this cycle. It's true some of the reactions to pain in our body are very hard to stop. We have no direct control over the effect of pain on our heart rate or blood pressure. This will happen automatically. We also have very little direct control over our feelings and emotions. It is extremely difficult to just decide you are not going let pain make you angry or depressed. However, we have a lot of control over our thoughts. Even though they may occur spontaneously, we are wired so that we can consciously control what we think. Certain thoughts may spring into our mind but we have the ability to create new, alternative ones.

This is reassuring. It means that we have the potential to break into this cycle of thoughts, feelings and pain and stop it. In fact, not only can we stop it, we can reverse it. If we can stop negative thoughts or replace them with good ones, it will feed back down the system in a good way. Positive thoughts will give rise to positive emotions, and positive emotions will have positive effects on the way our body functions. Finally, positive emotions will also have a helpful effect on the pain control centre, which will send messages down and close the gates and reduce our pain.

Retraining the brain: thought challenging

One way to use our thoughts to control our pain is by a process called thought challenging. This means that when negative thoughts come into our minds we don't accept them as necessarily true but challenge them. For example, if we experience a flare-up of pain, several thoughts may come into our minds such as: 'I must have re-injured myself', 'I am going down hill' or 'The pain is going to get worse'.

These thoughts are all understandable but negative and not necessarily true. You can challenge them by other thoughts such as: 'Pain doesn't always mean damage, it is most likely a flare-up', 'I know flare-ups don't last forever' and 'This pain will settle down again'. Simply challenging negative thoughts that are triggered by pain can be enough to block their negative effects on how we feel and how our body responds and can help to break the cycle of making the pain even worse. Thought challenging is like an anti-inflammatory for the mind!

'Thought challenging is like an anti-inflammatory for the mind!'

Retraining the brain: changing the way we think

Another way to change the way we think is through meditation. If thought challenging is like an anti-inflammatory for the mind, meditation is like a long-acting analgesic. Used regularly, it can have a powerful effect, even in small doses.

Meditation refers to a broad variety of practices much like the term sports. It means different things to different people. For some, meditation is a technique that promotes relaxation and well- being. For others, meditation is a deeper technique grounded in philosophies that require a certain religious or philosophical approach and often many hours of practice. Fortunately, you don't need to believe in a certain philosophy or learn a complicated technique to get the benefits of meditation.

At its heart, meditation is simply a technique that focuses the mind in a particular way in order to change thoughts, feelings and actions. One way of thinking about meditation is that its aim is to replace unhelpful thoughts with helpful thoughts. And changing thoughts is the key to changing feelings. Meditation then can be the key to using the power of our minds to overcome our pain and change the way we feel.

Meditation and pain

A number of studies now show that meditation is helpful for people with chronic pain.[1] [2] [3] One study looked at a group of people who regularly practised meditation and compared them with a group of people who did not practise meditation.[4] When they were given a painful stimulus to the skin, people who regularly practised meditation had an increased threshold for pain.

What is more interesting is that in this study, researchers also used a scanner to look at the brains of people who meditated and compared them with people who did not meditate. They found that people who meditated had thickening of the brain in areas that are involved in brain processing and this increased thickness was related to their lowered sensitivity to pain.

You may remember that we looked at how the brain is plastic or changeable and that we have the ability to affect this plasticity. Meditation is a technique that changes the brain and the way it responds by changing the way we think. There is now clear evidence that meditation has an effect on the brain and this is linked to a decreased sensitivity to pain.

Types of meditation

A widely practised technique is mindfulness meditation. It aims not only to make a person aware of thoughts and sensations but to let go of negative emotions that may be attached to that sensation. This means that even though a person is still aware of pain, the intensity and the suffering associated with the pain is reduced.

Another form of meditation is concentrative meditation. This involves focussing on a single word or phrase, the breath or an external object such as a candle or a leaf. It aims to help people rise above their normal feelings, thoughts and concerns by reaching a higher level of consciousness.

Many religious traditions have meditation as a fundamental practice. Although methods vary, generally in religious meditation, time is set aside to reflect on thoughts, feelings and actions and to draw closer to a higher power. This can be done through practices such as prayer and reflection on scriptures. One of the aims of religious meditation is to help connect with a higher power in a way that helps instil ways of thinking and acting that are in line with the core values of the religion, such as contentment and gratitude, as well as other qualities like compassion, patience and love.

To practise meditation, though, you do not need to use a particular technique or come from a religious background. Practising meditation

'Meditation is simply a technique that focuses the mind in a particular way in order to change thoughts, feelings and actions.'

can be as simple as spending some time thinking about certain experiences or reflecting on a piece of writing such as a poem or saying. As we have seen, the positive feelings that come from a time like this will flow down and be good for our body and good for our pain.

If you haven't practised meditation in the past, you may be feeling a bit uncertain about how to go about it or feel that it is going to be too hard or take up too much time. You may feel it just not for you. To help get you started, we will describe a couple of exercises that are very simple and have been shown to be helpful. Even if you are familiar with meditation, you may like to try them.

Gratitude exercise

1. Reflecting on experiences

○ This exercise can be done daily and need only take a few minutes. Find a quiet spot where you feel relaxed and not distracted. It may be a comfortable chair in a favourite spot, under a tree or lying in bed as you go to sleep.

○ Take a few minutes to think back over the day. Bring to mind something that you are thankful for. Spend a few seconds reflecting on it and enjoy the feeling of gratitude. You can be grateful for even the smallest things such as a smile, a beautiful flower, or a warm sunny day.

○ It may be helpful to write this experience down in a gratitude journal.

2. Reflecting on words

This exercise can be done on a daily or occasional basis. Turn to some inspiring words which encourage you to develop gratitude in your life. They may be a saying, a verse or a poem. Here are some examples but you may have your own:

Better to light one small candle than to curse the darkness.

Chinese Proverb

If the only prayer you ever say in your life is thank you, it will be enough.

Meister Eckhart (c. 1260-1327)

Sometimes our light goes out but is blown into flame by another human being. Each of us owes deepest thanks to those who have rekindled this light.

Albert Schweitzer

Wake at dawn with a winged heart and give thanks for another day of loving.

Kahlil Gibran

Spend some time reflecting on these words and contemplate their meaning for you.

Gratitude—Making it part of your life

Decide when you will meditate

○ An important step in making gratitude part of your life is to find a regular time for a gratitude exercise. Once you have found something that works for you, try to find a regular time when you can practise it. As a minimum, once a week is generally recommended to get the most effect. But two or three times each week would be even better!

○ The time does not have to be long. If you are doing it on a regular basis, five minutes is enough to start changing the way you feel. You may also like to include it as part of your relaxation technique.

Have a plan to maintain this new skill

As with the other skills that we have explored so far, any technique will only work for as long as we maintain it. Use a similar approach to help maintain it as a regular practice:

○ Have a concrete plan—write down when you are going to meditate. If it is a regular time such as each night before you go to sleep or each Sunday evening after dinner, this makes it easier to remember and make part of your life.

○ Be accountable—get a friend to check how you are going on a semi-regular basis.

○ Mix it up. It's good to learn and become skilled in one technique of meditation. However some people find it helpful to use more than one approach for variety and to keep their times of meditation fresh. Feel free to explore different techniques and to change them from time to time.

Finally, you may choose to share these feelings of gratitude. In reflecting on people or things you are thankful for, you may want to tell someone and let others share the same feelings. You may wish to call someone, email or write to them and tell them how you are thankful for what they have done or who they are. Gratitude shared has a multiplying effect on you and others!

Summing up

Gratitude is extremely important in living with pain. It may counteract the effect of stress and pain in our lives and can help us overcome feelings like anger and sadness. No matter what we are facing, regular times of meditation where we build attitudes of acceptance, contentment and gratitude can help us cope better, live happier and healthier lives and reduce pain. Take some time now to work out how you are going to build acceptance and gratitude into your life.

Fact file: Gratitude

- Our thoughts have a large influence on our feelings

- Our feelings have a large influence on the part of the brain that controls our pain.

- Building positive thoughts creates positive feelings which help reduce pain

- Gratitude is an attitude that has been shown to have positive effects on how we feel

- We can build gratitude by taking time to be thankful.

Chapter 8

Step 4—Courage

*I am 85 and fractured my hip in a fall. I needed a lot of
courage just to get on my feet again. The pain and fear
of falling could have disabled me but I didn't let it.*

Ruth, music teacher

The problem of fear

We react to pain with fear, which is a useful and even necessary reaction to things that hurt us. However, over the long term, it can make life worse for the person with chronic pain. It may not only directly increase pain but also indirectly increase pain by decreasing activity and adding to deconditioning.

Fear adds to pain in several ways. It can help to create the state of hypervigilance, which we looked at earlier. As we described, hypervigilance is like having a highly tuned internal radar that is constantly scanning and looking for harmful information. This means that people who are hypervigilant are extremely alert to any potentially harmful signals from the body. This opens the spinal gate and turns up the volume of pain and other incoming signals so that there is a heightened sensitivity to pain.

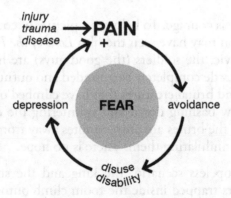

An additional factor that can add to fear and make our pain worse is another process we looked at earlier: catastrophising.[1] People in this situation not only fear, but fear the worst. For the person with chronic pain, they can become convinced that anything they attempt will have disastrous consequences. Catastrophising is closely linked to hypervigilance and again makes our body more sensitive to pain. Dealing with both of these is an important part of overcoming our fear and reducing pain.

Fear and avoidance

If we experience pain when we move a certain way, it doesn't take our minds or our bodies long to realise that this movement will very likely cause us pain the next time. And once we make that connection, we become fearful of it happening again.

In acute situations, this is very helpful. It is a tremendously useful reaction that protects us from all sorts of danger and harm. However, fear does not serve us as well in the long term. People with chronic pain often react in the same way as if they have acute pain. They stop what they are doing to minimise the pain. After a while, they will not even try, because they know it will bring on the pain.

Although this is a natural and understandable reaction, it is not helpful. If it continues, it will make our pain worse. If a person stops doing something that causes pain, they become less active. And as we saw before, the less active we are, the more deconditioned we become. And the more deconditioned we are, the worse our pain becomes.

Overcoming fear: courage

The way past fear is courage. To help get a picture of courage, let's go to the movies. You may have seen the film *Lord of the Rings*. At one point in this movie, the soldiers (the good guys) are holed up in a small room in a castle completely surrounded and outnumbered by a vast sea of ugly and brutal creatures that have climbed over the castle walls and are now bashing down and splintering the door of their room. You know the brutes are only minutes away from charging in and completely annihilating them. There is no hope.

Facing this hopeless scenario, the king and the small band of remaining soldiers trapped inside the room climb onto their horses. Then with a loud shout from the king, they lift their swords and charge out of the room through the splintered door and into the swirling mob to what looks like certain doom.

'To move forward and do things in the face of pain requires courage.'

This scene captures the attitude that is so important in learning to overcome our pain—courage. Not the absence of fear, but the ability to overcome fear and charge forward even though the odds are overwhelming. To move forward and do things in the face of pain requires courage.

Courage is required to go for a walk when we know it is going to result in more pain for the rest of the day and possibly for the rest of the week. Courage is required to exercise when we know we have a weakness in a disc in our back that we are worried may give out and cause even more problems. Courage is just as important in fighting pain as it is in facing an army of ugly brutes bent on destroying us.

The first response to pain is fear—to withdraw. Courage is not the absence of fear. It is a miracle fibre within you—a little voice that says I will get up and try tomorrow.

John, age 30, paraplegic from sporting accident

The benefits of courage

Researchers have found that courage is one of the key characteristics of people who are hardy or resilient. Such people are able to face stressful circumstances such as pain and turn them to their advantage and even into opportunities for growth.

This ability to face difficult circumstances in a positive way does not come easily or naturally and our upbringing has a large effect on our ability to cope with fear and stress. However, no matter what our upbringing or age, it is a quality that can be learned and developed.

In addition, courage is a quality that feeds on itself. When you face a challenge that scares you, it leads to a sense of achievement and satisfaction that can make you keener to take further steps of courage.

Courage is not only good for us; it is good for those around us. People who are courageous are more likely to look outside themselves and respond to the needs of others. Courage enables people to go beyond just coping to fully embracing and enjoying life, to reach out despite their hurt and fear and give to others.

Courage and pain

Courage not only has general benefits in making us feel better but it also helps our pain. As we have seen, avoidance leads not only to physical deconditioning but also to depression through lack of exercise, poor sleep, loss of relationships and the benefits for our minds of doing things that bring enjoyment and satisfaction.

Courage is important in overcoming pain. It helps us to conquer fear and take on activities that we may be afraid will cause us damage or increased pain. And as we increase our activities, we will reduce deconditioning, make ourselves fitter and give ourselves other benefits that come from being more active.[2]

Linda's story—a story of courage

Linda, a brown-eyed mother of three young children worked as an ambulance driver and also volunteered as a fire-fighter with her husband, although one parent always stayed home with the children. During a long hot summer Linda went with a team of fellow volunteers to fight a bushfire. The team was faced quite suddenly with a fire that burned out of control, fanned by a sudden change of wind.

'Courage is not only good for us; it is good for those around us.'

The team's vehicle was hit by a falling tree and as Linda struggled to help move the vehicle, she slipped and fell under the back wheels just as it became free. Linda's legs were badly crushed and though her life was spared she spent months in a rehabilitation clinic learning to walk again. But she was left with severe chronic pain and was unable to return to her old job. She became depressed, began drinking and smoking marijuana to try to cope with her pain and her sense that her life had lost meaning. Formerly a loving wife and mother she became too despondent to care for her family. The situation became so bad that her husband eventually told her that unless she began to change her ways, he would leave her and take the children with him.

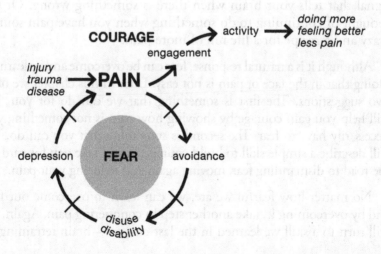

Linda was shocked, but decided she would try to find ways to cope with her pain. An opportunity to teach disabled children to swim came along and Linda, with some self-doubt, saw this as a wake-up call. She saw the enthusiasm of the disabled children as they struggled to learn to swim and began to gain hope. After some time,

Linda decided to train as a swimming coach, and after many months as a coach found that she had begun to regain strength in her legs and that her pain, although still present, had decreased with exercise. She had learned to cope not only with her pain and disability, but also with her feelings that life had lost meaning. She returned to study, qualified as a medical records technician, and now works in the medical record department at her local hospital.

For Linda, courage was the key to breaking out of the cycle of pain, fear and diminishing activity. Linda realised that she was going to lose everything including the people she loved if she continued down the path of trying to deaden her pain through self-medicating. She chose to face her fears with courage. As a result, she is now doing more, feeling better and has less pain. She found her life again.

How to build courage

Fear and avoidance are both natural and deeply inbuilt responses to pain. We may realise that fear is stopping us from doing things and making our pain worse. But fear is so ingrained that it can seem impossible to overcome. Either you may not want to overcome it or feel that you cannot. You may still be convinced that pain is a useful signal that tells your brain when there is something wrong. Or the thought of continuing to do something when you have pain sounds crazy and a recipe for a life full of more pain.

Although it is a natural response, fear can be overcome and unlearned. Doing that in the face of pain is not easy. Later in this chapter we offer two suggestions. The first is something that we can do for you. We will help you gain courage by showing how pain is not something you necessarily have to fear. The second is something that you can do. We will describe a simple skill to build courage. It will take you forward on the road to dismantling fear, moving again and reducing your pain.

No matter how fearful we are, we can learn to overcome our fear and by overcoming it, take another step in conquering pain. Again, we will turn to a skill we learned in the last chapter—brain retraining or

'No matter how fearful we are, we can learn to overcome our fear and by overcoming it, take another step in conquering pain.'

thought management. The big step in unlearning fear is to unlearn a message that we feel instinctively: that pain is telling us that something is wrong. The message that we want to get across strongly is this: pain does not always signal damage. As we shall see, pain can be due to changes in the nervous system and can also be part of the healing process. Let's look a bit more closely at both of these facts.

Pain can be due to changes in the nervous system

The first fact is that chronic pain has more to do with what is happening in our nervous system than in our bones, joints or wherever the pain is coming from. With acute pain, it is usually the case that pain is very much related to damage. If you have a tooth abscess or appendicitis, nerves signal that damage is happening or about to happen. It is right to seek immediate treatment.

However with chronic pain, the situation is quite different. As we saw in the chapter that looked at how pain works, the nervous system changes when you have had pain for any length of time. Chronic pain winds up and sensitises the nervous system. This means that the nervous system turns up the volume on messages coming from your body. If you become hypervigilant or are catastrophising, this turns up the volume even more and the pain can be unbearable even though the signals are not that big.

For example, a person who has had low back pain for several years may get severe pain when they bend or move. Investigations may show that there are some changes in the discs or joints but no major damage to give rise to severe pain. The pain is coming from the discs and joints. But the volume of the messages is turned up so that by the time they reach the brain they are far stronger and the pain is severe. This means that the pain is way out of proportion to what is happening in our body. The brain then is giving us false information.

This does not mean that the pain is not real or even not severe. What it does mean is that the severity of the pain does not reflect the amount of damage, nor does it signal that we are causing damage by moving. We have no need to fear what our brain is telling us.

Pain can be part of the healing process

The second fact is that pain can be part of the normal healing process. If you have participated in sport or done something strenuous for the first time like climbing a steep hill, you know afterwards that you experience pain. Your muscles and joints can ache, sometimes for days.

This pain that we experience after intense exercise is a natural response to increased activity. It does not signal damage. There may be some inflammation but this is not damage. It is part of the body's response to intense activity and in fact is an important response that helps us on the path to becoming fitter.

The problem for most people with chronic pain is that they have become deconditioned. If pain has made you inactive for any length of time, your muscles, ligaments and joins will lack condition. They will be unfamiliar with working hard. Like the athlete who experiences pain on their first workout of the season, any increase in activity will result in pain. If you add in some central sensitisation, the pain can be severe.

The important thing to remember is that while the pain may be severe, it is not signalling damage. It is the normal response of muscle, joints and ligaments to activity after a period of inactivity. What is more, it is a positive sign that the body is reacting in a way that is moving towards being fitter. There is no need to be fearful.

'Each time we ignore the voice of fear and do something, we become just a little stronger.'

Dismantling fear

The best pain control technique of all was my own determination that I would not let pain take over my life.

Pain may be a part of life, but it is not all of it.

Rob, age 72, retired motor mechanic

Pain, and even severe pain, does not always signal damage. Chronic pain sensitises the nervous system so that messages are amplified and pain can be the normal response of your body to increasing activity.

This is all very well. But it doesn't get around the fact that the pain still hurts. If you have chronic pain, chances are that doing things makes your pain worse. You may understand that it is not necessarily a sign of damage, but this doesn't get around the fact that it still hurts. How can you get past your pain and your fear of it hurting to do more?

This is the next step in building courage and it is something that you can do. We should warn you that there is no simple one-step procedure to getting rid of your fear. However, there is a simple skill that you can practise, which builds on what you have learned about damage. This skill will help your mind and body unlearn the connection between fear and damage, increase your fitness and help reduce your pain.

It will take some time, especially if you are very fearful. However, even the most fearful person can use this skill to gradually decrease their fear levels and get back into life. Let 's look at the next steps in overcoming fear.

Don't listen, just do

The first step, as we have seen, is to pay less attention to what our bodies are telling us. This may sound difficult when your body is in severe pain. However, your pain is like a demanding child wanting to get attention and making all sorts of threats if you don't do what they say.

To get around this and to reduce the power of the demands, refuse to listen. If you remind yourself that the pain is not a sign of damage and therefore you don't need to respond, it will take away a little of the power of the demand to stop. Each time you tell yourself this and each time you do something despite the pain, the demands will lessen. Gradually, you will weaken the fear and weaken the strength of the demands. You will find that you have greater strength to ignore what those voices inside are saying.

The second step is to just do it. Each time we give in to the voice of fear and avoid doing something we become just a little weaker. On the other hand, each time we ignore the voice of fear and do something, we become just a little stronger.

What we do does not have to be big. In fact, it is better if it is not too big. But taking a step against our fear is a step in the right direction. This is courage. You may not feel very courageous and even the smallest step may seem huge and even insurmountable. So let's look at a practical way to build courage and do things in the face of fear.

Pain, fear and graded exposure

One way to face fear and build courage is a technique used by clinical psychologists called **graded exposure**. This technique involves making a conscious decision to face situations that normally make you fearful but in a controlled and graded way. For example, if you have a fear of spiders, it may be a bit much to suggest that you overcome your fear by just sticking your hand into a jar of spiders!

'Chronic pain has trained your brain to be more and more fearful and more and more sensitised to pain. Graded exposure is a way of reversing this.'

However, you may have enough courage to touch a plastic spider. You could then play with it and handle it. You may then have enough courage to touch a sealed container with a spider inside. You may then touch a very small spider that is known to be safe. You may then allow a small spider to crawl over your hand.

As you can see, in this approach of graded exposure, the aim is to gradually increase the danger stimulus and allow yourself to come to terms with a level of discomfort that you can manage. Studies have shown that this approach is tremendously effective in helping people with fear and pain to do more. In fact, one study compared two groups of people with chronic low back pain. One group was taught the technique of graded exposure. The other group had a back operation; a spinal fusion. At the end of the study, they found that the group who had learned the technique of graded exposure and used this to increase their activity levels improved just as much as the group that had an operation.

The other advantage of graded exposure is that it retrains your brain. Unfortunately, chronic pain has trained your brain to be more and more fearful and more and more sensitised to pain. Graded exposure is a way of reversing this. Each time you do something in the face of pain you retrain your brain to realise that doing something may increase your pain but it won't harm you. And as the fear of harm lessens, so will your pain.

Meditation and courage

I migrated to Australia from Eastern Europe and some years before arriving in Australia I developed severe, intermittent abdominal pain. The pain frightened me as it was apparently related to previous surgery and I was told that no cure was known. I came to believe that my pain would eventually kill me and I lived in such fear that I often spent sleepless nights. I was taught meditation and during this I remembered the courage I'd once shown when saving my brother from drowning. I made courage a focus during meditation practice. As I continued this daily practice, courage seemed to expand and grow, and my fear of pain and death diminished. Then I added a graded exposure to pain so that I could focus on the pain without fear, increasing this pain exposure a little each day. In time I was able to manage my pain successfully. It's still a presence in my life, but with meditation it seemed to lessen and to lose its control over how I feel, and I was able to sleep!

Helen, age 48

In the previous chapter, we looked at meditation as a skill that can help build acceptance and gratitude with beneficial effects that flow through to help our pain. Meditation can also be a way to build courage through dealing with fear or anxiety and will add further to improving the way you feel and reducing your pain.

We have already looked at using the time of meditation as an opportunity to reflect on negative feelings such as sadness, anger or fear and to move forward toward acceptance and gratitude. However, in that meditation exercise, we did little to address fear.

In order to do this, we will add another component to your time of meditation. As you take some time to focus on things that you are thankful for, also spend some time dealing with your fears and anxieties. In fact, we would suggest that you do this before moving on to the time of being thankful.

It will not be possible to deal with all the anxiety and fears that may be present. You may like to focus on one that comes to the top of your mind. Again recognise and acknowledge the fear or anxiety and the impact it is having on you.

Then, spend some time to think on the resources you have to overcome this fear. This may be your own internal strengths. It may also be sources of strength outside you such as family, friends, health professionals, community, writings or a higher power.

Spend some time reflecting on the resources you have available and how they may help you face your fear with courage. This may mean spending some part of your meditation time in reading or prayer. It may also mean making a decision to draw on some of these resources at a later time in order to help you overcome your fear.

Courage—making it part of your life

How then do we make courage a part of who we are? First, we find those situations that require courage. If you have pain, you probably don't have to look far. Any situation or activity that causes pain requires courage. Once you have done that, there are several steps that you can take to build courage.

Decide what you are going to do that requires courage

○ Choose an activity that you would like to do but currently don't do because you are worried that it will either cause damage or increase your pain.

○ If you are uncertain, consult with your health practitioner and check whether what you propose to do involves a high risk of doing harm. Any activity involves risk and most activities will cause pain. So remember that no one can guarantee that you won't be harmed. You are not asking whether it is likely to increase your pain. You are asking whether they feel the activity is likely to be safe.

Decide how you are going to tackle it

○ Once the level of risk has been clarified, plan how you are going to engage in the activity. Try to find a bite-sized, achievable chunk that requires some courage but does not completely terrify you.

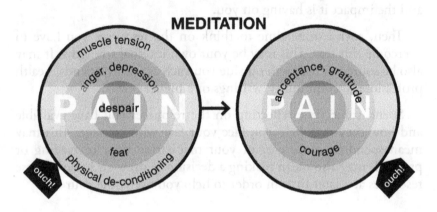

Find activities and resources that give you courage

○ Make your times of meditation an opportunity to foster and build courage.

○ Find a friend or a family member who can help you face your fear and encourage you to push through with the challenge you have set yourself. Tell them that you want to do something that needs courage but you need their help to do it. You will be surprised how many people will line up to help, because other people love being around courage—it makes them feel good.

○ Spend time around people who are courageous and you will become courageous too. Learn what makes them tick and let their courage rub off on you. Meet them, listen to them, read books, watch movies and listen to stories about people who are courageous. Use their courage to inspire you.

○ Find a support group to give you courage. A group that exhibits courage and encourages you to do the same would be ideal. A good group will challenge you through their words and their example. They will help to give you the strength to be courageous and do things that you didn't think you were capable of doing.

○ Tell your health practitioner you would like to step out and do more but are fearful. Set some guidelines with them and get their support.

Just do it!

○ Once you have made a plan and have resources in place to help, go ahead—just do it.

○ If you have asked a friend to be there and help give you courage, get them to come along as well.

Enjoy the moment

○ Once you have completed the task, bask in the moment and enjoy the feeling of overcoming your fear.

○ You may like to share with a friend, health professional or support group what you have done.

Keep it going

○ Take time to congratulate yourself for what you have done and be thankful to whoever helped you be courageous. You may even like celebrate in a small way—buying yourself a small treat, having dinner at a nice restaurant or doing something else that gives you pleasure.

○ Keep growing in courage—plan your next challenge!

Summing up

Courage helps counteract the harmful effect of fear and avoidance that pain produces in our lives. Courage will make us stronger in both body and mind. Take some time out now to work out how you are going to build courage into your life.

God, grant me the serenity to accept

the things I cannot change,

the courage to change the things I can,

and the wisdom to know the difference.

Fact file: Courage

- Pain can lead to fear avoidance.

- Fear avoidance can result in physical and mental deconditioning.

- Courage enables us to overcome fear and face new challenges.

- Accomplishing new things not only makes us physically stronger but makes us feel good.

- Courage comes from understanding how pain works.

- Courage grows by taking small steps of risk.

Chapter 9

Step 5—Hope

Shannon's story

At the age of 22, Shannon, a high school graduate who worked as a secretary, developed a severe pelvic pain condition. Her pain was so severe that she found it difficult to complete a demanding work day, and her social life became almost non-existent.

Shannon experienced what many who suffer from chronic pain find—that pain is invisible. Her work colleagues could not understand why Shannon could barely manage to end the workday without extreme fatigue and sometimes, an irritable mood. Her friends were unable to recognise that she could not go to concerts, stay out late at night, and attend parties without excusing herself and going home. Shannon began to lose confidence in her abilities when, despite surgery, her condition did not improve. She became sad and depressed, and lost hope in her ability to manage her life and her pain.

After a long period of struggle, Shannon, who had always loved art and music, decided that she would leave her job and study art. She had some savings, and with trepidation enrolled in an arts program. She found that studying art played to her strengths, was what she loved doing and gave her life a new sense of meaning and purpose.

The importance of hope

For many, chronic pain can lead to despair. The antidote to despair is hope. Hope is crucial not only for the enjoyment of life but for survival. Viktor Frankl, a Jewish psychiatrist and neurologist, was working in Austria at the outbreak of the Second World War and was imprisoned in a concentration camp. Frankl wrote about the importance of hope.

In the camp, Frankl was confronted by incredible suffering. However, he was amazed at the ability of some people to withstand the suffering they all faced. What he noticed was that those prisoners who lost hope were those who often did not survive. On the other hand, the people who were able to find some kind of meaning in what they faced were able to endure horrendous suffering.

Frankl survived the camp and in 1946, after his release, wrote and published a book called *Man's Search for Meaning*[1]. In this book, he writes:

The prisoner who had lost faith in the future—his future—was doomed. With his loss of belief in the future, he also lost his spiritual hold; he let himself decline and became subject to mental and physical decay. Usually this happened quite suddenly, in the form of a crisis, the symptoms of which were familiar to the experienced camp inmate. We all feared this moment—not for ourselves, which would have been pointless, but for our friends. Usually it began with the prisoner refusing one morning to get dressed and wash or to go out on the parade grounds. No entreaties, no blows, no threats had any effect. He just lay there, hardly moving. If this crisis was brought about by an illness, he refused to be taken to the sick-bay or to do anything to help himself. He simply gave up. There he remained, lying in his own excreta, and nothing bothered him anymore.

Hope is crucial. Without hope, life becomes intolerable and unliveable. With hope, people can show incredible courage and strength in the face of almost unbelievable hurt and suffering. Finding hope is a vital element in facing pain and finding life.

Real hope and false hope

How though do we find hope? It is all very well to say that we need hope to overcome pain but how do we do it? Many people look to health professionals for hope. Understandably, they want them to say that they can do something that will get rid of their pain or make it a lot better. And, just as understandably, health professionals long to bring people this kind of hope. They want to be able to tell someone that they have discovered the cause of their pain and that they have something that will take it away.

However, very often getting rid of chronic pain is just not possible. As we have seen earlier, it is very difficult and sometimes impossible to be sure what is causing pain. And, even if we have a good idea of what is causing it, more often than not we are unable to relieve it completely.

The person then who offers the hope of getting rid of pain in this situation is dishonest and unhelpful. The person in pain is often desperate for hope and the health professional, even with the best of intentions, is keen to provide it. However, telling someone that they can be helped when it is most likely that their pain will continue is unfair. Such a promise is false hope.

'Telling someone that they can be helped when it is most likely that their pain will continue is unfair.'

It feels good for a time but the person becomes even more disappointed when he or she finds that what was promised cannot be delivered. False hope increases despair.

Offering real hope

People with pain need realistic hope. But if it is not hope of getting rid of pain, what hope can we offer? Viktor Frankl recognised the importance of finding hope but it would have been false hope to tell people in the concentration camp that they would certainly survive or that the war would soon be over.

Instead, Frankl said the way forward to finding hope was to change the nature of the hope. And this changing of hope was to somehow find meaning in the midst of suffering.

The question is: How do we find meaning in the middle of pain or suffering? Is it trying to find out why you are in pain so that you understand why it is happening? Or is it trying to find the answer to the meaning of life when you have back pain? These sorts of questions can sound impossible to answer and completely irrelevant in helping to deal with pain.

If we are to believe that finding meaning is going to have any benefits and if we are going to put it into practice, it would be helpful to know exactly what we are talking about. Before we go further then, let's look at what we mean by meaning.

The meaning of the message

Meaning can have three aspects that we will explore here further. The first is fairly superficial and is simply the meaning of the message. It is trying to figure out what something indicates or signifies. For example, the letters C-O-W when put together signify an animal with four legs that stands in a field and gives us milk. Or a loud voice coming from a face that is tight and red with one extended finger pointing in my direction may indicate that I have done something wrong.

In these situations, we work out what things mean on the basis of the information we receive. We then react, based on that information. The important thing for us is that our reaction is based on our interpretation of the information.

What has this to do with pain? This type of meaning is very important. The way that we react to pain is very much determined by how we interpret the message and the way we think about pain. As we saw in the chapter on courage, if we interpret pain messages as damage, if that is the meaning that it has for us, then we are likely to react by withdrawing and avoiding. Re-interpreting the meaning of the message is another aspect of retraining the brain.

But our interpretation of the pain is crucial in how we respond and deal with it. Awareness that pain does not necessarily signal damage is an important step in treating pain.

The meaning of the pain

I got my finger caught in the car door. The top of it had to be amputated. I did not feel pain until I got to the hospital and realised that I would lose the top of my finger. At that moment the pain was overwhelming, intolerable even with strong medication. I was a concert pianist. I realised that I may not play the piano again. This was my life. Playing the piano gave my life meaning. Eventually the tissues in my finger healed but the pain in my finger continues to this day.

Susie, aged 29, concert pianist

Pain is much more than a message that is received by our brains and may very well be signalling something other than damage. This is extremely important knowledge in helping to reduce pain and its impact on how we feel. But the pain may still be present. So where does meaning come in then?

Another aspect of meaning is not so much what the pain signals but what it means for my life. For example, bright red tongues of flame jumping from the roof of my house with large red trucks, men in large hats and hoses all around it may signal that my house is on fire. This is what the messages mean. At a deeper level, this may mean that I need to find somewhere else to stay for the night or even that I am ruined because I was not insured and my life savings were poured into the house. These meanings can have an impact from as little as finding somewhere else to stay to facing financial ruin.

This sort of meaning is also crucial to our experience of pain. Continuing pain may make it difficult to work so that, like the person whose house burnt down, your whole financial future is looking uncertain. Or it may make it difficult to play with the grandchildren. Instead of a retirement where you can enjoy getting to know them and play with them, you may feel that your relationship with the grandchildren will never be what you wanted.

In these situations, pain does not just signal damage to your body, it signals damage to your life. And the more damage to your life that you believe the pain signals, the more distressed you will be. If you believe that pain has ruined your life so that there is nothing to look forward to, it is very likely that you will feel little motivation, drive, enthusiasm or energy for anything. Your spirit will be crushed.

Changing the meaning of the pain

To change these effects, one of the things that we can do is to change the meaning of the pain. By this we don't mean finding the answer to why you are suffering. Nor are we suggesting that you must see the pain as good rather than bad. It is changing the meaning of the pain so that it is no longer simply something that has ruined your life.

Changing this meaning requires us to look at our lives and find those things that are still good despite the pain. It is not saying that the pain has not affected our lives nor even had a major impact. But it is looking within the suffering to find which parts of our lives still contain things that give us enjoyment and pleasure.

If we can do that, we can change the meaning of the pain so that it is no longer something that has destroyed or ruined our lives. Instead, life still contains things that we enjoy and can continue to enjoy into the future. When we identify these things, we can move from the despair of a ruined life to the hope of a life that contains something positive. And when our mood and thoughts are more positive, this changes the way our brain functions and helps to close the gates that may have opened and increased the levels of pain.

We know that this is not easy. As we have already seen, the impact of pain is severe and deep and in no way do we want to diminish that. For many people with pain, it is very difficult to believe that life contains much, if any, good either now or in the future. When you are faced with pain that has caused so much hurt and damage it can seem hard or impossible to see anything positive.

However, your ability to enjoy life in the presence of pain depends strongly on how well you can do this. The more you can see past the pain and see things that you still enjoy and that still give you pleasure, the greater your ability to change the meaning of pain for your life. And the more you can change the meaning of pain, the better your life will be.

Daniel's story

Daniel is someone who came to see Rebecca about his pain. He was a successful builder, happily married with three children. In January 2003, his life changed dramatically when he fell from a building he was working on, damaged his spine and was left paralysed. Daniel was unable to walk and for much of his rehabilitation, Daniel suffered with feelings of anger and immense loss. For the first two months in the spinal unit, he continued to question the point of going on. In 2006, Rebecca received a letter from Daniel, which simply said:

> Thanks for walking those dark months with me in the rehab unit and for continually encouraging and believing in me when life was at its darkest point. I have grown to realize that my horrible accident took my legs away but it didn't take my spirit away. I have learned that I am much more than my pain. There was no magic bullet. I needed to reinvent myself in order to continue what I enjoyed most. I have become more human. I am more in touch with what really matters in life.

'We can change the meaning of
the pain so that it is no longer
something that has destroyed
or ruined our lives.'

The meaning of life

The next aspect of finding meaning goes beyond our pain. It is
finding meaning in life. It is more closely linked to words like purpose
and is about finding things in our lives that give us meaning and
direction. Most of us don't think in those terms and talking about
finding meaning in life may sound a bit abstract or heavy. The fact
is, whether we think about it in those terms or not, all of us find
meaning in life in some way.

Another way to look at the concept of meaning is to think about
things that you feel are important or are your priorities. For example,
if you were to list the most important things in your life, they may be
your family and your work. If these are the things that are important
to you, your priorities are usually set around them. They will be
things that you pour time and energy into. They are the things that
for you make life meaningful and enjoyable.

The Japanese people have a word that captures this concept:
ikigai. It is often difficult to translate a word such as this adequately,
but it contains the idea of those things that make life worth living,
that give a person hope and motivation and that make life purposeful
and meaningful. In its simplest form, ikigai is described as having
something to get up for in the morning. Studies of the people of
Okinawa in Japan have found that ikigai is a key characteristic of
these people who are amongst the longest living on the planet.

Pain can obviously affect our sense of meaning and purpose in life. If pain prevents us from enjoying the things that are important to us, then it is going to make our lives worse. And the more things that it seems to interrupt and the more strongly it interrupts them, the worse our lives will be. If pain prevents us from doing all the things that were really important to us, then life can seem meaningless and without purpose. And, once this happens, there can be little drive, energy or pleasure in life.

Finding meaning in life

My friend Jan was dying of breast cancer at home. She was not really a spiritual person but she had a purpose in her dying—it is hard to explain but her dying had a profound effect on everyone around her. She decided to die as she had lived. Her home became a stream of love. Her good friends cooked food and came over—there was plenty of laughter and joy amidst the pain. I look back on this time with Jan and feel that it was sacred time. Her dying had a huge impact on me.

Jenny, age 43, artist and good friend of Jan

The way to recover meaning in life in the face of pain is to re-evaluate our priorities and to see if we can find enjoyment in things that were unimportant or overlooked before. For example, some people with cancer who have no hope of recovery still find meaning in life. Simple objects of beauty, nature, or relationships that have been restored and deepened can become a new source of enjoyment.

Part of this may not only be having new priorities that give us a greater appreciation for things around us. We may develop new priorities that give us a greater appreciation for things around us. We may also discover a new purpose that gives our life meaning through what we do. Many people who have experienced suffering re-evaluate their priorities and decide to live their lives differently with a new perspective and purpose.

'As much as we may resent or hate it, pain can be the stimulus to re-evaluate who we are and where our life is going.'

As we have seen, pain can rob us of the things that we enjoy so that we have nothing to look forward to. We may feel that life is meaningless as long as we continue to suffer. To counter this feeling, we need to find something that still brings meaning and purpose to our life. No matter what we can't do because of our pain, we need to find something we can do that brings a sense of meaning and makes life fulfilling and enjoyable.

If you have chronic pain, you face the real possibility of ongoing pain that is difficult to get rid of or even reduce substantially. The challenge then is to be able to extract meaning and hope from the suffering. To quote Viktor Frankl again:

> We must never forget that we may also find meaning in life even when confronted with a hopeless situation, when facing a fate that cannot be changed. For what then matters is to.... transform a personal tragedy into a triumph, to turn one's predicament into a human achievement. When we are no longer able to change a situation—just think of an incurable disease such as inoperable cancer—we are challenged to change ourselves.

Pain as a catalyst for change

This quote from Viktor Frankl leads us to our last point on finding hope and that is through change. There is no doubt that chronic pain can affect us terribly. In no way do we want to downplay or appear to diminish the suffering that pain can bring. If there is any chance of taking away pain or reducing it, of course that should be done.

However, pain can be an opportunity for change. As much as we may resent or hate it, pain can be the stimulus to re-evaluate who we are and where our life is going. As Frankl says, 'we are challenged to change ourselves'.

Many people travel through life with very little reflection. Some of us only give much thought to life when things get tough toward the end. It is then that people often start to reflect that, if they had their time over again, they would have lived with different priorities and with a different perspective on life. In fact, many cancer survivors live with a whole new perspective on life that is clearer to them than before.

Pain and suffering can force us to look at where we are going and how we are living our lives. Pain may have closed some doors or made old ones seem unattractive. The secret of continuing to live life with vitality and passion in the face of pain is to find new sources and new things to live for. This is why people who live with pain and suffering often have a depth of understanding and wisdom that others lack. They see things with a clarity that others miss and have developed priorities that are different.

To help illustrate this, we turn to an article written by Dr Robert Mack in the New England Journal of Medicine some years ago. Dr Mack was a successful surgeon who was diagnosed with advanced cancer. He says:

> It became poignantly clear to me… that this was a time of real choice. I could sit back and let my disease and my treatment take their course, or I could pause, and look at my life and ask, 'What are my priorities? How do I want to spend the time that is left?'. One of the really ironic things about the human experience is that many of us have to face pain or injury or even the possibility of death in order to learn the real purpose of being and how best to live a rewarding life.[2]

Pain then, rather than being a disaster that ruins our life, can be an opportunity and a catalyst for change and for growth. Hard as it may be to accept, many people find that, although pain may be resented at first, it forces them to change, and to change for good.

Pain, meaning and hope

At the beginning of this chapter we talked about hope—both false hope and real hope. It is very easy to lose hope when we have chronic pain. It is easy to pin all our hope on getting rid of the pain or at least finding something that will take away most of it. We can become convinced that this is the only thing that will make life enjoyable again.

Finding meaning offers the possibility of becoming hopeful without necessarily getting rid of the pain. It does not rule out the hope that the pain may go away or be relieved. But it changes the way that we view the pain and the way we view our life so that we can move past the pain and find enjoyment.

Finding meaning, then, helps to give us hope in three ways. First, it gives us hope by realising that pain doesn't necessarily mean damage. This frees us to move forward without the fear of causing further harm. Second, it gives us hope by recognising that the experience of pain is not completely negative. Even in the midst of pain there have been some positive things that we have learnt or can still enjoy. And third, finding meaning gives us hope by finding things in life that we can still look forward to. It is finding that there are things that we can still enjoy that bring purpose and meaning to life.

Finding meaning and purpose: Life reflection

So how can we find meaning and build hope? Questions of meaning and purpose are not simple or superficial. They require some thought and reflection. Even if we are willing to consider it, taking time out from our busy lives just to think can seem difficult or a waste of time. Let us look a bit further at the nature of reflection.

Reflection has been defined as 'exploring our experiences in order to lead to a new understanding and appreciation.' This means that reflection is not just sitting down and gazing at our navel or trying to dig deep into our thoughts. It is looking at our experiences so that we can change and move forward with a new plan of action. It is examining where we are and what we are going through and how we might change so that life is richer and fuller.

This extended time of reflection and dealing with thoughts and feelings in a deep way in order to move forward in life can be highly effective in facing not just physical pain but also deep hurt and

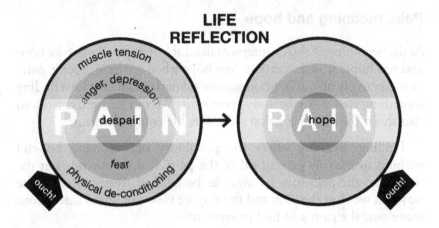

LIFE REFLECTION

muscle tension

anger, depression

despair

PAIN

fear

physical de-conditioning

ouch!

PAIN

hope

ouch!

suffering. These reflective times help in finding healing and release and in moving forward with new life-giving qualities. You may like to explore the possibility of taking some extended time for life reflection. Although it may sound demanding, many people have found giving time to reflection hugely helpful, not just for dealing with pain, but for getting the most out of life no matter what their situation.

Reflection then, far from being difficult or a waste of time can be one of the most productive and life changing of experiences. Through reflection, it is possible to find new energy, new motivation, new meaning and new purpose. It is about restoring hope by looking at our lives and reconnecting with those things that bring energy, passion and fun. It is another crucial ingredient in facing pain and finding hope.

Hope—Making it part of life

Decide how you are going to do it

○ If you haven't engaged in reflection as a way of building hope, or have not done so since your pain began, set aside a time for reflection. It may seem strange or difficult to find time for this. However, regaining a sense of hope, meaning and purpose in your life doesn't happen in a few minutes. You may like to schedule an hour or even a half-day.

- You may like to get away to new surroundings away from the normal pressures and busyness of life so that you are free from distractions.

- It may be helpful to do this with a friend, mentor or spiritual guide. They can be useful to provide some direction and a sounding board. Choose someone whom you trust and who understands what you have been through and where you are going.

During the time of reflection

During the time of reflection, consider and reflect on what has been happening to you during the past 12 months or longer. You may want to make notes, writing things down. Here are some questions to guide your thinking:

- What has happened to me over the last year (for example, experiences, events and relationships, good and bad)?

- What was important to me before my pain started? Which of these has been affected by pain? Have my priorities changed since the pain? Are some things more important or less important?

- What can I still enjoy despite my pain? What do I come away from feeling energised and uplifted? What things, activities or relationships do I really enjoy and find important to me? What would I do with my time if pain and money were not an issue?

- Are there things that I want to change or do differently (for example, change my activities, relationships, priorities)?

- How will I do that? What is my plan?

After the time of reflection

- You may want to talk these things over with someone close to you.

- Look at how you can put your plan into action. If it requires help, courage or support, enlist the help of those who can assist you put your plan into effect.

- You may find it helpful to have a time of reflection regularly. In 12 months, re-evaluate and see how things have gone.

Summing up

Finding meaning is a crucial step in recovering energy, drive and zest for life. No matter what damage pain has done in our lives, finding out what is important to us, what gives meaning and purpose to our lives and what drives and motivates us can be the key to being re-energised and finding new hope and enjoyment in life.

Fact file: Hope

- Pain can lead to loss of hope and a crushed spirit.

- Loss of hope comes through loss of meaning and purpose in life.

- Rediscovering meaning and purpose can lead to renewed hope.

- Hope revives and strengthens the spirit.

- Meaning, purpose and hope can be rediscovered through life reflection.

Chapter 10

Living with hope

Lin's Story

Attached to Philip's pin board in his office is an inspiring letter. It is from the husband of a woman named Lin, whom he saw in the Pain Management Centre. Not long before coming to the Centre, she had a malignant lump found in one breast and ended up having both breasts removed. Sadly, like many people following this type of operation, she was now suffering from severe, shooting nerve pain over the upper part of the chest and was looking for something to help the pain.

During the next few months, the pain management team and her oncologist tried various options to help her. It was not possible to get rid of her pain but they gradually settled on a combination of gabapentin (an anticonvulsant medication that helps some people with nerve pain) and a transcutaneous electrical nerve stimulator (TENS machine), as well as learning some skills in pain management.

These options helped and they were able to reduce her pain a little although it was still quite severe. Despite helping her to some degree, one of the most significant things was not what they did for Lin but what she did for herself. Following her diagnosis, she decided she was going to make the most of whatever time she had left. She had a husband, children and grandchildren and she was going to do as much as she could for as long as she could, pain or no pain. And she did just that. Here is part of the letter that her husband sent to Philip several years after her first visit:

Dear Professor Siddall

The purpose of this letter is to express our thanks to you and the whole Pain Management team.

It is now four years since Lin first visited the clinic. Our experience during our just completed holiday in Africa and Madagascar highlighted to us just how much had been achieved since May 2004.

As examples I attach three photos. One of Lin sleeping out under the stars in the middle of the salt pans of the Kalahari Desert, another is of wild Kalahari Desert meerkats using us as high sentinel lookout points and a third is of Lin with lemurs in Madagascar. Four years ago we would not have believed such experiences to be possible.

Lin of course, still has very significant pain and cannot do without the mitigation of gabapentin and her TENS machine. Just as important has been the psychological lessons learned from the personal care at the clinic and from the pain management book, combined with Lin's determination to get on with life.

In your professional field I am sure that you have many successes and some disappointments. Both Lin and I are very grateful that you have made it possible for her to have a full life, despite her pain.

Thank you once again.

Engaging with life

Lin's story is an example of many things that we have talked about in this book and it leads us into our last chapter: Living with hope. Lin is a remarkable woman, although she would not see herself that way. Even though she had been given a diagnosis of cancer and continued to experience severe pain, she made a conscious decision with her husband to live life to the full in the remaining time that they had. She was not going to let the pain stop her.

Finding hope in the face of pain was not solely due to mind over matter. She did not decide that the pain was in her mind and she would simply grit her teeth and bear it and make do as best she could. Overcoming her pain meant using a combination of treatments that helped to reduce her pain as much as possible. These treatments included medications and a stimulation technique. She also took up Tai Chi, painting and ikebana which she found helped her to relax. Even though she still felt significant pain, the relief was important for her. She remained active with her week full of constant engagements and activities.

Acceptance, gratitude and courage were also important ingredients of her life. She accepted both her pain and her diagnosis of cancer. This did not mean that she did not wish that the pain would go away or that she was happy at the thought of leaving her family. Instead, she acknowledged that both had affected her life. However, she did not spend all her time or energy focussing on making them go away or wishing they had never happened. Instead, once she was satisfied that she had received good advice and appropriate treatment, she decided to move forward and make the most of her life.

Lin also showed thankfulness for all that she had. Although she had been diagnosed with cancer and the treatment had left her with severe ongoing pain, she was thankful for her supportive husband, her children and grandchildren and the activities that she could still enjoy.

Lin was a woman of courage. She decided to change some of her activities to allow more time for relaxation. And, she decided that, rather than cocoon herself, she would try to engage with life despite the pain. It did not stop her from trips in the desert sleeping on a camp bed.

Lin also found hope. Despite a diagnosis of cancer and the presence of pain, she reflected on those things that gave her meaning and purpose and made a concrete plan to make them part of her life and enjoy them as much as possible.

Lastly, she built partnerships that supported her but also challenged her to live life to the full. These included our centre, her local doctor, her husband and family. These partnerships were more about helping Lin to do as much as she could and get the most out of life rather than trying to get rid of her pain. Although she was always keen to reduce her pain if possible, she accepted that we had done as much as we could and would keep looking for any new treatments that came along.

Finding hope

Lin is an example of someone who has faced pain and found hope—even when it hurts. However, every person's story is different. Every person in pain faces different struggles, different challenges and different fears. Whatever is causing you pain and whatever its impact, your life will be better if you put into practice the skills you have learned in this book. These include skills that will reduce the tension that can build up in your body, the deconditioning that results from doing less, the anger, depression and fear that comes from dealing with constant pain and the despair that can come from the prospect of ongoing pain that no-one can fix.

Together, these skills will make you more relaxed, stronger, calmer, happier, and ultimately you will experience less pain. All of this will enable you to reclaim your life and rediscover the things that bring enjoyment and pleasure.

A life with hope

As we come toward the end of this book, the message we hope you take away is that, no matter what you are facing, pain does not have to dominate your life. Far from it! There are skills that you can learn and attitudes that you can develop that can actually turn pain from something that has the potential to ruin your life into something that can be a catalyst for change and growth. It can help you to re-evaluate where you are going and who you are.

And, if you put into practice the skills that we have introduced in this book, they will help your pain, and build strength in body, mind and spirit. It is our hope that they will enable you to face the future with greater confidence in your ability to manage your pain, with hopefulness for what lies ahead.

Professor Phil Siddall
Rebecca McCabe
Dr Robin Murray

June 2013

Further Reading

Chapter 1 – Understanding pain

1. Graven-Nielsen T, Sörensen J, Henriksson KG, Bengtsson M, Arendt-Nielsen L. Central hyperexcitability in fibromyalgia. Journal of Musculoskeletal Pain 1999;7(1-2):261-271.

Chapter 2 – How does pain work?

1. Woolf CJ, Ma Q. Nociceptors—noxious stimulus detectors. Neuron 2007;55(3):353-364.

2. Lee M, Tracey I. Unravelling the Mystery of Pain, Suffering, and Relief with Brain Imaging. Current Pain and Headache Reports 2010;14(2):124-131.

3. Beecher HK. Pain in men wounded in battle. Annals of Surgery 1946;123(1):96-105.

4. Melzack R, Wall PD. Pain mechanisms: a new theory. Science 1965;150:971-979.

5. Woolf CJ. Central sensitization: Implications for the diagnosis and treatment of pain. Pain 2010;152(3, Suppl. 1):S2-S15.

6. Norman Doidge The Brain That Changes: Itself Stories of Personal Triumph from the Frontiers of Brain Science, 2007, Penguin, New York.

7. Peper E, Wilson VE, Gunkelman J, Kawakami M, Sata M, Barton W, Johnston J. Tongue Piercing by a Yogi: QEEG Observations. Applied Psychophysiology and Biofeedback 2006;31(4):331-338.

Chapter 3 – How does pain affect us?

1. Indo Y, Tsuruta M, Hayashida Y, Karim MA, Ohta K, Kawano T, Mitsubuchi H, Tonoki H, Awaya Y, Matsuda I. Mutations in the TrkA/NGF receptor gene in patients with congenital insensitivity to pain with anhidrosis. Nature Genetics 1996;13:485-488.

2. Cox JJ, Reimann F, Nicholas AK, Thornton G, Roberts E, Springell K, Karbani G, Jafri H, Mannan J, Raashid Y, Al-Gazali L, Hamamy H, Valente EM, Gorman S, Williams R, McHale DP, Wood JN, Gribble FM, Woods CG. An SCN9A channelopathy causes congenital inability to experience pain. Nature 2006;444(7121):894-898.

Chapter 5 – Relaxation

1. Kubota K, Tamura K, Take H, Kurabayashi H, Mori M, Shirakura T. Dependence on very hot hot-spring bathing in a refractory case of atopic dermatitis. Journal of Medicine 1994;25(5):333-336.

2. Anonymous. Integration of behavioural and relaxation approaches into the treatment of chronic pain and insomnia: NIH technology assessment panel on integration of behavioural and relaxation approaches into the treatment of chronic pain and insomnia. Journal of the American Medical Association 1996;276(4):313-318.

3. Carroll D, Seers K. Relaxation for the relief of chronic pain: a systematic review. Journal of Advanced Nursing 1998;27(3):476-487.

4. Cepeda MS, Carr DB, Lau J, Alvarez H. Music for pain relief. Cochrane Database of Systematic Reviews 2007;3:3.

5. Roehrs T, Hyde M, Blaisdell B, Greenwald M, Roth T. Sleep loss and REM sleep loss are hyperalgesic. Sleep 2006;29:145-151.

6. Chiu YH, Silman AJ, Macfarlane GJ, Ray D, Gupta A, Dickens C, Morriss R, McBeth J. Poor sleep and depression are independently associated with a reduced pain threshold. Results of a population based study. Pain 2005;115:316-321.

Chapter 6 – Exercise

1. Brown AK, Liu-Ambrose T, Tate R, Lord S. The Effect of Group-Based Exercise on Cognitive Performance and Mood in Seniors Residing in Intermediate Care and Self-Care Retirement Facilities: A Randomized Controlled Trial. Br J Sports Med 2009;43:608-614.

2. Sullivan A, Scheman J, Venesy D, Davin S. The role of exercise and types of exercise in the rehabilitation of chronic pain: specific or nonspecific benefits. Current Pain and Headache Reports 2012;16:153-161.

3. Sullivan AB, Covington E, Scheman J. Immediate Benefits of a Brief 10-Minute Exercise Protocol in a Chronic Pain Population: A Pilot Study. Pain Medicine 2010;11:524-529.

4. de Meirleir K, Naaktgeboren N, Van Steirteghem A, Gorus F, Olbrecht J, Block P. Beta-endorphin and ACTH levels in peripheral blood during and after aerobic and anaerobic exercise. European Journal of Applied Physiology & Occupational Physiology 1986;55:5-8.

5. Berger B, Owen D. Mood alteration with yoga and swimming: aerobic exercise may not be necessary. Percept Mot Skills 1992;75:1331-1343.

Chapter 7 – Gratitude

1. Kabat-Zinn J, Lipworth L, Burney R. The clinical use of mindfulness meditation for the self-regulation of chronic pain. Journal of Behavioural Medicine 1985;8:163-190.

2. Teixeira ME. Meditation as an intervention for chronic pain: an integrative review. Holistic Nursing Practice 2008;22(4):225-234.

3. Morone NE, Lynch CS, Greco CM, Tindle HA, Weiner DK. I Felt Like a New Person. The Effects of Mindfulness Meditation on Older Adults With Chronic Pain: Qualitative Narrative Analysis of Diary Entries. The Journal of Pain 2008;9(9):841-848.

4. Grant JA, Courtemanche J, Duerden EG, Duncan GH, Rainville P. Cortical thickness and pain sensitivity in Zen meditators. Emotion 2010;10:43-53.

Chapter 8 – Courage

1. Vase L, Nikolajsen L, Christensen B, Egsgaard LL, Arendt-Nielsen L, Svensson P, Staehelin Jensen T. Cognitive-emotional sensitization contributes to wind-up-like pain in phantom limb pain patients. Pain 2011;152:157-162.

2. Brox JI, Storheim K, Grotle M, Tveito TH, Indahl A, Eriksen HR. Evidence-informed management of chronic low back pain with back schools, brief education, and fear-avoidance training. Spine; 2008;8:28-39.

Chapter 9 - Hope

1. Frankl, V. (2006). Man's Search for Meaning. Boston: Beacon Press.

2. Mack, R. M. (1986). Lessons from living with cancer. New England Journal of Medicine, 311, 1640-1644.

Acknowledgements

The authors would like to thank and acknowledge the many people whose conversations, ideas and feedback have contributed to this book.

We are thankful to family and friends who provided encouragement, support, and advice at different stages and who helped shape and form the book. In particular, Phil would like to thank his wife Rhonda, who helped create the spark that set this book in motion. We would also like to thank Grace Tague, Linda Critchley, Ali Asghari and Trudy Maunsell from Royal North Shore Hospital Pain Management and Research Centre, Sydney. It was their invaluable input and stimulating discussion that helped crystallise our unformed ideas and guide this book from vague theories to a concrete reality.

Thanks to Paul Monkerud, Ilsa Neicinieks, Pauline Smith and Philippa Jones who read various sections of the manuscript and offered valuable insights and advice.

We would like to thank Ivor Indyk and Anne Deveson whose feedback was not only hugely helpful in the writing of the book but whose professional advice and warm encouragement was instrumental in steering us through the mysterious world of writing and publishing.

Our editor Rosie Scott did an excellent job of taking our writing and expertly and supportively moulding the text towards its final form. Although she should not take the blame for its shortcomings, it would not have been the book it is without her insights and suggestions. Coralie Wales and others at Chronic Pain Australia and Elizabeth Carrigan of the Australian Pain Management Association also provided helpful feedback and criticism of the book and their input and suggestions were very much appreciated.

Peter Hallett and Richard Knight from HammondCare have been excellent midwives in the final stages of getting this book to publication. Not only have they been a pleasure to work with, but their encouragement, enthusiasm for the project and expert guidance in editing and thinking through the design and presentation of this book took away any pains of gestation.

A special thanks to the Sisters of Mercy Parramatta for their generous support.

Finally, we would like to thank the senior management at HammondCare. Their support for the ideas in this book in many different ways has enabled us to translate words into action and allowed us to bring to life our own dreams and hopes.

Appendix

the pain book
extra

The Pain Book authors Philip, Rebecca and Robin recommend these additional practical techniques, activities and exercises.

Special relaxation for headaches

This relaxation technique involves special considerations for those who suffer either migraines or tension-type headaches, or both. It combines progressive muscle relaxation with a visualisation technique developed by psychiatrist, Milton Erickson.

It is a technique that you can call into play when a headache begins to develop.

Imagine a scale graded from one to 10. Decide where your headache falls on this scale. For example, a really bad headache might be a 'nine'; a lesser headache might suggest a measure of 'four' or 'five'.

Begin by finding yourself a quiet place, and sit comfortably (or lie down), then begin breathing gently and rhythmically. Now take yourself through the progressive muscle relaxation.

When you have completed the progressive muscle relaxation, focus on your hands, and notice that they are becoming warmer-you may even imagine gloves making them feel warmer. Focus now on your feet, and notice they are becoming warmer, perhaps you may wish to visualise socks warming them up.

Now, with your eyes closed, imagine yourself walking toward a beautiful lake. As you move toward the lake, envision a beautiful, peaceful scene. In your mind's eye, see yourself resting comfortably on soft grass by the side of the lake. Again, in your imagination, see that the clouds have formed a number that is the measure you have given your headache. Let's say you have decided on a 'six'. As you watch the clouds in the form of a six, let them slowly change and re-shape themselves into a five. While you are watching, notice that you are breathing gently, rhythmically, and softly. As you continue watching the clouds, they gently re-shape themselves into a four, then a three. Notice your hands and feet remain warm, but that a gentle cool breeze has begun to circulate around your head, so that your head is becoming cooler. As you watch the clouds, they gradually form into a two, and then drift down toward the lake. The cloud settles on the lake and then takes the form of a swan gently gliding across the lake. You notice that your head feels cool, your hands and feet warm and you feel completely relaxed as you continue breathing gently.

Stretching program

**Recommended by author Rebecca McCabe –
Senior Physiotherapist**

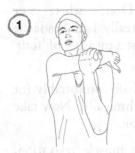

1 Stand or sit.

Stretch one arm over to the opposite shoulder by pushing it at the elbow with your other arm. Hold the stretching about 15 seconds. Relax.

Repeat two times.

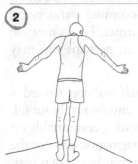

2 Stand in a corner of a room, facing the corner. Lift both arms to horizontal position against the walls.

Let your upper trunk lean into the corner until you feel the stretching of your chest muscles. Stretch about 15 seconds.

Repeat two times.

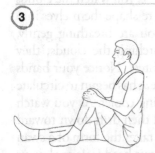

3 Sit on the floor with one leg straight and the other bent with your arms around it.

Try to straighten your bent leg while resisting any movement with your arms for five seconds. Relax. Then pull the leg closer to your body. Hold about 15 seconds.

Repeat two times.

4

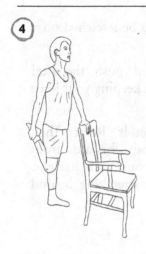

Stand holding on to a support with one hand and to the ankle with the other hand.

Pull the ankle towards your bottom, then try to straighten the knee for about 15–30 seconds while resisting with your hand.

Relax your leg and repeat the exercise pulling the ankle a little bit further. Return to starting position.

Repeat two times.

5

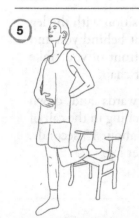

Stand straight with one knee bent and supported on a chair.

Tighten your buttock muscles and straighten your hip.

Tighten your stomach muscles, do not let your back arch.

Hold 15–30 seconds.

Repeat two times.

6

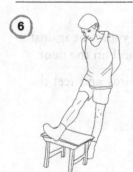

Stand with the leg to be stretched on a chair, heel over the edge.

Push the opposite hip forwards and bend your trunk forwards keeping your back straight. Hold about 15 seconds.

Repeat two times.

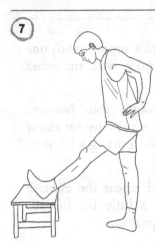

7

Stand with the leg to be stretched on a footstool.

Flex your ankle and push the heel towards the footstool keeping your knee straight.

Hold about 15 seconds. Relax. Then bend your upper body forwards from your hips keeping your back straight. You should feel the stretching behind your knee and thigh.

Repeat two times.

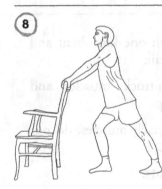

8

Stand in a walking position with the leg to be stretched straight behind you and the other leg bent in front of you. Take support from a wall or chair.

Lean your body forwards and down until you feel the stretching in the calf of the straight leg. Hold about 15 seconds. Relax. Stretch the other leg.

Repeat two times.

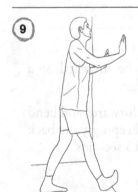

9

Stand facing a wall. Put your foot against the wall keeping your heel on the floor.

Bring your pelvis forwards and feel the stretch in your calf.

Repeat two times.

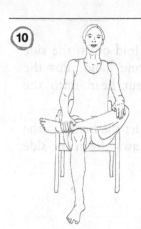

10

Sitting on a chair with your foot on the opposite knee.

Gently push your knee towards the floor.

Repeat two times.

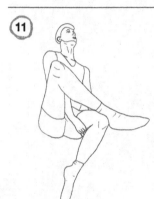

11

Lying on your back with knees bent. Cross the ankle of the leg to be stretched over the other knee. Put your arms around the thigh as shown.

Bring your thigh towards your stomach. Feel the stretch in your buttock.

Repeat two times.

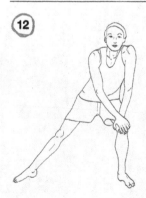

12

Stand with legs astride and straight.

Bend one leg and put your hands on the knee. Bend your leg even more and put more weight on the leg. You will feel stretching on the inside of the thigh on the straight leg. Hold about 15 seconds.

Repeat two times.

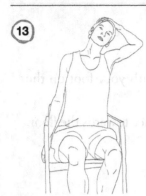

13

Sitting on a chair. Hold on to the side of the chair with one hand. Put the other hand over your head onto the opposite ear.

Tilt your trunk and let the hand on the ear bend your head away from the side to be stretched.

Repeat two times.

'Stretching is an extremely valuable skill in treating chronic pain. If you have pain, it is almost certain that surrounding muscles have tightened as a natural reaction to protect the body.'

Tai Chi—18 Movements

Recommended by Rebecca McCabe

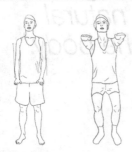

1 Waving hands by the lake

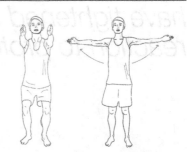

2 Expanding chest on top on top of the mountain

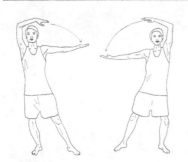

3 Painting the rainbow

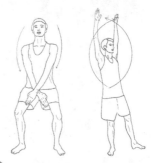

4 Parting the clouds

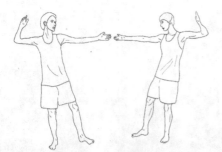

5 Weaving silk in the air

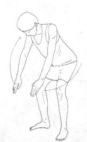

6 Rowing the boat

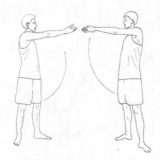

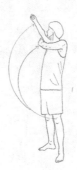

7 Sage presents peach

8 Gaze at the moon

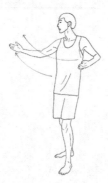

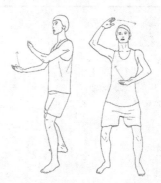

8 Wind rustles Lotus leaves

10 Waving hands in the clouds

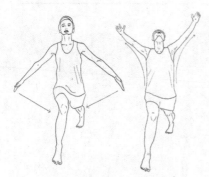

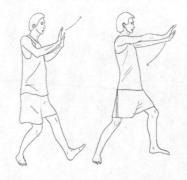

11 Scooping the sea and viewing the sky

12 Rolling with the waves

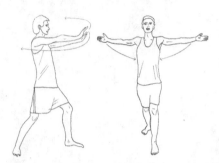
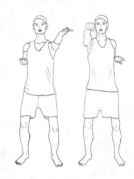

13 The dove spreads its wings

14 Dragon emerging from the sea

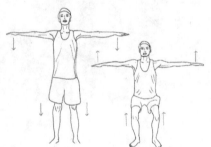
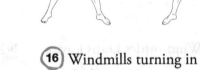

15 The flying wild goose

16 Windmills turning in the breeze

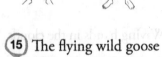
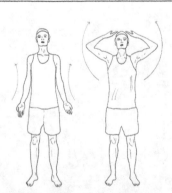
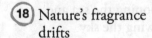

17 Bouncing ball in the sunshine

18 Nature's fragrance drifts

Strength Training Exercises

This section on strength-training is adapted by Rebecca McCabe from materials developed by Professor Maria A Fiatarone Singh, MD, FRACP— Fit for Your Life Foundation Ltd—and used with her kind permission.

Tips for your strength training program

○ With each lift (repetition) inhale before you start to lift the weight, then exhale as you start to lift it (breathe out on the effort). Never hold your breath while lifting the weights. Take a full breath in and out before starting the next lift. Allow two to three seconds of rest between each lift.

○ For the best results, choose a range of exercises that use all the major muscles groups of your arms, legs and trunk.

○ For gaining muscle strength, lifting weights is better than pushing against an object.

○ Always do the movement slowly, through the full range of motion as possible for you. Take about six–nine seconds for each movement, spending equal time lifting the weight as you do lowering it. Alternate between your left and right arms and legs, allowing one set of muscles to rest while the others are working.

○ Never swing the weight or use momentum to help you lift it. Follow the method shown in the pictures later in this section to avoid injury.

○ It is important to keep the correct posture when you do any lifting activity, to protect your back and neck and work the muscles correctly. A simple way to do this is to pull your belly button in towards your spine. When you do this it should not be so hard that it stops your breathing - it should feel like a slight tension in your abdominal area.

○ Before adding any weights to your arms or legs test the muscle group by slowly and carefully performing one or two lifts through the full range of motion. If you have increased pain when you do this you should check with your doctor of physiotherapist before going further. If you can't do a whole set of eight lifts with no weights without becoming tired or fatigued, just practice until you can. Then you can begin to add weights.

○ During the first two weeks, warm up to an amount of weight that feels hard to lift but which you can lift eight times the proper way before having a rest. For example, if you have chosen 2.5kg weights but you find you get too tired after six lifts, use only 1-2kg to start with. Starting at a weight that is too light just means it will take a few more sessions to reach your goal. Starting with a weight that is too heavy could cause injury, so stay on the side of safety to start with.

○ Your goal is to do two or three sets of eight to 12 lifts with the weight you have chosen. Remember to rest each muscle group for one or two minutes between sets. Do not increase the weight until you can do the two or three sets in a single session. You can either do one set of each exercise, then go back to the beginning and repeat the cycle, or you can do two to three sets in a row with a rest period in between.

○ As soon as the weight that you are lifting for two to three sets no longer feels as hard as it did to start with, increase the amount of weight for that exercise. This is the most important point for effective strength training. The exact amount of increase will be different for each person. Increasing by a small amount each session (0.5–1kg) is better than increasing by large amounts intermittently. Each time, your goal is to do two or three sets of eight to 12 lifts with a weight that feels hard to lift.

○ Exercise two to three days a week. Do not exercise the same muscle group two days in a row. Your muscles need a day off between training sessions to recover. However, it is fine to exercise your arms one day and your legs the next day if you find that you are tiring when doing them both in a single session

○ You can expect in the early stages of training to feel delayed muscle soreness one or two days after a training session. This is part of the process of muscle rebuilding and repair which ultimately leads to larger and stronger muscles. It feels like a mild ache or tenderness in the muscles you have exercised, but is not sharp and it doesn't stop you from being able to get around. It feels strongest about two days after the exercise session, and will happen less and less as you train regularly.

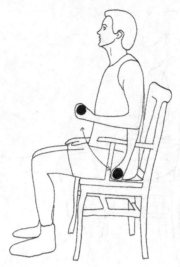

(1) Biceps curls

This exercise will strengthen the upper arm muscles which flex the elbow.

1. Sit erect with your arms at your sides, holding the dumbbells.

2. Bend one arm at the elbow to lift the dumbbell toward your shoulder. Don't move the upper arm or shoulder during the lift.

3. Lower the dumbbell slowly to the starting position.

4. Repeat with your other arm. Alternate arms between each lift or lift both arms at the same time.

Tips

Remember: breathe out on the effort.

Don't lift the weight by moving your shoulder and upper arm. Keep your elbow flexed at your side.

Don't arch your back when lifting the dumbbell.

Don't slouch or move your elbow forward during the lift.

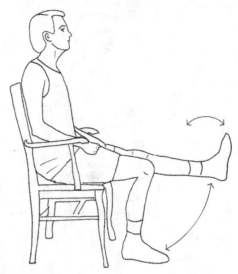

② Knee extensors

This exercise will strengthen the quadriceps muscle at the front of the thigh which straightens the knee.

1. Sit erect in a chair with the back of your knees resting against the chair seat and the weights strapped around your ankles.

2. Raise one foot in front of you until your knee is as straight as possible.

3. At the top of each lift, pull your toes back towards your head as far as possible, hold for five seconds, and then point the toes.

4. Lower your leg slowly to the starting position.

5. Repeat, alternating legs between lifts.

Tips

- Remember: breathe out on the effort.

- If you have knee problems, extend only as far as comfortable, otherwise try to completely extend the knee if possible.

- Sit all the way back in the chair, don't slouch or arch your back during the lift.

- If needed, insert a rolled towel under your knees so that your foot clears the ground during the lift.

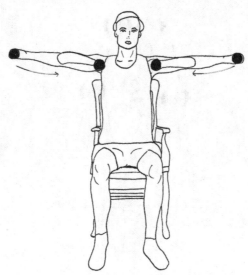

③ Triceps

This exercise will strengthen the muscles at the back of the upper arm which straighten out the elbow.

1. Sit erect in a chair holding the dumbbells horizontally just in front of your chest, with your elbows pointing out to the side.

2. Keeping the weights parallel to the floor, straighten out your elbows fully.

3. Bend your elbows to slowly return the weights to the starting position.

4. Repeat.

Tips

○ Remember: breathe out on the effort.

○ Don't let the weights travel down towards the floor.

○ Keep your elbows up throughout the movement.

○ Don't move your back or upper body, except for your forearms.

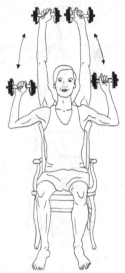

④ Overhead press

This exercise will strengthen the muscles of the shoulder and the back of the upper arm, which allow you to reach overhead.

1. Sit erect in a chair holding the dumbbells at shoulder level with palms facing forward.

2. Slowly lift both arms straight overhead until your elbows are straight and the dumbbells are touching, directly over your head.

3. Lower the dumbbells following the same path, and repeat.

4 The dumbbells can rest in your lap between repetitions as needed.

Tips

○ Remember: breathe out on the effort.

○ Relax your shoulders.

○ Don't arch your back during the lift.

○ Don't lift the weights in front of your chest and face.

○ Weights should be held shoulder-width apart during the lift.

○ Don't turn your palms inward during the lifting or lowering of the weights.

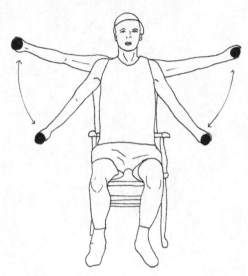

⑤ Side shoulder raises

This exercise will strengthen the shoulder muscles that lift the arms out to the side.

1. Sit erect with your arms hanging by your sides, holding a dumbbell in each hand with your palms facing your body.

2. Slowly raise both arms, keeping elbows straight, until your arms are parallel with the ground.

3. If one or both shoulders are limited by pain or stiffness, lift the arm as high as it will go without discomfort.

4. Slowly lower your arms back to the starting position.

Tips

- Remember: breathe out on the effort.
- Relax your shoulders.
- Don't use your back to lift the weight or arch your back during the lift.
- Don't swing the dumbbells up.
- Don't lift your arms higher than shoulder level.
- Don't turn your palms outwards during the lift.

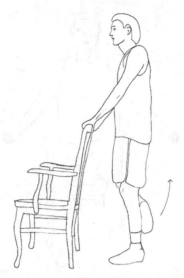

(6) Plantar flexors

This exercise will strengthen the ankle and the muscles in the calf.

1. Stand erect, holding onto the back of a chair, with ankle weights in place

2. Raise your body up as high as possible on your toes, without letting go of the chair.

3. Lower your body slowly to the starting position.

4. When this is too easy, lift your body weight using only one leg at a time, alternating right and left legs.

Tips

○ Remember: breathe out on the effort.

○ Alternative (as shown in the picture) -

○ Lift one foot slightly off the floor or hold it around your other ankle, and raise and lower your body using only one leg.

○ Alternate legs between sets.

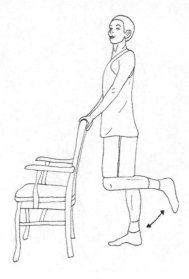

⑦ Knee flexors

This exercise will strengthen the hamstring muscles in the back of the thigh, which bend the knee.

1. Stand erect, holding onto the back of a chair, with ankle weights in place. Leave very little space between your body and the back of the chair.

2. Without moving your upper leg at all, bend one knee so that your heel is as close to the back of your thigh as possible.

3. Lower your leg to the starting position and repeat with alternating legs.

Tips

- Remember: breathe out on the effort.

- Don't move your thigh or bring your knee forward during the lift. Keep your knees aligned and just lift the lower part of your leg so the foot is as close to the thigh as possible.

- Don't bend forwards at the waist during the lift

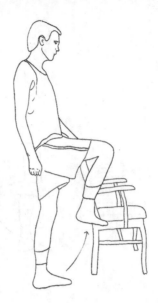

(8) Hip flexors

This exercise will strengthen the muscles that bring the knee towards the chest.

1. Stand next to a chair, holding onto the back of the chair, with ankle weights in place.

2. Without bending at the waist or letting go of the chair, bring one knee at a time as close to your chest as possible.

3. Lower to the starting position and repeat, alternating legs.

Tips

○ Remember breathe out on the effort.

○ If one chair is not enough support, stand between two chairs, holding onto each char with one hand.

○ Don't bend at the waist.

○ Bring your leg as close to your chest as possible.

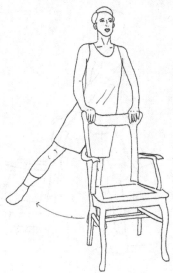

⑨ Hip abductors

This exercise will strengthen the muscles at the side of the hips and thighs, which pull your legs out to the side.

1. Stand erect, holding onto the back of the chair, with ankle weights in place.

2. Without bending your knee or waist, move one leg straight out to the side, making sure that your toes are always pointing forward.

3. Lower your leg to the starting position and repeat with alternating legs.

Tips

  Remember: breathe out on the effort.

  Don't point your toe out to the side during the lift.

  Don t bend at the waist or move your upper body during the lift.

  Keep your knee straight as your leg goes out to the side.

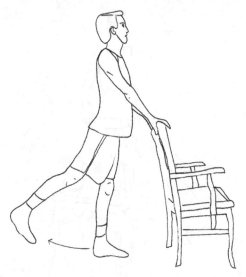

(10) Hip extensors

This exercise will strengthen the muscles of the buttocks and lower back.

1. Stand holding onto the back of the chair and bend forward about 45O at the waist, with ankle weights in place.

2. Lift one leg straight out behind you as high as possible, without bending your knee or moving your upper body.

3. Lower your leg to the starting position and repeat with alternating legs.

Tips

Remember: breathe out on the effort.

Don't bend your knee as you lift your leg out behind you.

Don't move your chest towards the chair as you attempt to lift your leg Keep your upper body stationary during the lift.

Don't arch your back during the lift or go so high as to cause back pain.

Index

Greenwich Hospital Pain Clinic

The Pain Clinic at Greenwich Hospital in Sydney provides treatment for people with chronic non-cancer pain and cancer survivors with chronic pain.

The clinic is comprised of a multidisciplinary team of health professionals and seeks to help people by providing careful assessment and appropriate treatment tailored to individual circumstances. The treatments offered are designed to reduce pain and help with other aspects of life that are affected by pain, including things like physical activities and mood. The clinic provides:

○ Medical management including the use of pain relieving medications

○ Referral for appropriate interventions when indicated

○ Physiotherapy including exercise instruction and functional rehabilitation

○ Hydrotherapy

○ Clinical psychology including personal instruction in pain management skills

○ A multidisciplinary group pain program

For more information email **painclinic@hammond.com.au**

Other HammondPress pain resources

Pain in older people and people with dementia: A practice guide ($24.95). Pain can be hard to recognise and manage in older people and people with dementia, especially when communication is limited. This book by expert Dr William McClean offers insight into best practice in pain management, and is full of practical and easily applied strategies for supporting the care of older people and people with dementia.

www.dementiacentre.com.au

The Authors

Professor Philip Siddall is a specialist pain medicine physician and Director of the Pain Management Service at Greenwich Hospital in Sydney, Australia. He has been working in the field of pain management for more than 25 years and previously worked at the Pain Management Centres at Royal North Shore and Royal Prince Alfred Hospitals, Sydney as well as Addenbrooke's Hospital in Cambridge, England. He is conjoint Professor in Pain Medicine at the University of Sydney and enjoys teaching students and health professionals from a range of disciplines. He is an active researcher and recognised internationally for his work in the field of pain management with many publications in scientific and medical journals, regular invitations to speak at national and international meetings and for six years he was the Australasian representative on the international council of the International Association for the Study of Pain.

Rebecca McCabe is the senior physiotherapist of the Pain Management Service at Greenwich Hospital in Sydney. She is President of the Bethany Health Care Centre in Strathfield, a multidisciplinary facility, and has undertaken research at the Royal North Shore Pain Institute, into the effectiveness of a self–management program to help older people cope with pain. This research was published in the journal Pain. As a member of the Sisters of Mercy, Parramatta, Rebecca has spent most of her working life committed to assisting people in pain. In her younger days, Rebecca represented Australia as a swimmer.

Dr Robin Murray is a clinical psychologist and neuropsychologist with 20 years of experience in the practice of psychology, and 13 years in pain management at Royal North Shore Hospital and Canberra Hospital. She now works in the Pain Management Service at Greenwich Hospital. Dr Murray trained as a clinician in San Francisco, USA. She has worked as an international trainer in the Psychology of Happiness and in the Management of Chronic Pain and has completed research projects related to chronic pain. She is also experienced in the treatment of depression, the management of work-related difficulties, and in helping people relate to each other in ways that enhance growth.